JOB BURNOUT
IN
PUBLIC EDUCATION

**Symptoms, Causes,
and Survival Skills**

JOB BURNOUT
IN
PUBLIC EDUCATION

Symptoms, Causes, and Survival Skills

Anthony J. Cedoline
Director of Pupil Services
Oak Grove School District
San Jose, California

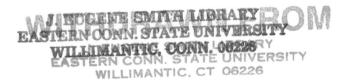
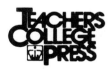
Teachers College, Columbia University
New York / London   1982

Published by Teachers College Press, 1234 Amsterdam Avenue,
New York, N.Y. 10027
Copyright © 1982 by Teachers College, Columbia University

Library of Congress Cataloging in Publication Data

Cedoline, Anthony J.
  Job burnout in public education.

  Bibliography: p.
  Includes index.
  1. Teachers—Job stress.   2.   School administrators—Psychology.
3. Burn out (Psychology)   I.   Title.
LB2840.2.C425   371.1′001′9   81–23289
                                        AACR2

ISBN 0–8077–2694–X

Manufactured in the United States of America

87 86 85 84 83 82   1 2 3 4 5 6

Contents

Acknowledgments

Grateful acknowledgment is due to each author whose research and scientific investigation have provided the foundation for this volume. Special thanks go to Rose Noack and Jim Hastings for their assistance in the preparation and editing of this book. In addition, I extend my appreciation to my wife Clare and children, Maria, Antonia, and Peter, whose tolerance and understanding exceeded my obliviousness to their needs. Finally, many thanks to the Oak Grove School District for providing me with a sabbatical leave, making this book possible.

Prologue: Age of Anxiety

In April 1979, the *Wall Street Journal* ran a series of articles entitled "The Age of Anxiety." The findings indicated that stress is an acute and increasing problem for Americans. The chairman of the University of Chicago's psychiatry department was quoted as saying, "I doubt if the people of other times had the information overload that we have." The following studies were reported:

Item: A nationwide sampling of 2,500 people by the National Institute of Mental Health found that 27 percent had experienced high levels of distress during the year prior to the interview. Two social psychiatrists uncovered ten "life strains" that are linked with a significant degree of anxiety and depression—five related to occupation, three to marriage, and two to parenthood.

Item: Results of a 1976 study of emotions were compared to those of an identical survey taken 20 years earlier. The 1976 survey found that 13 percent of those surveyed were unhappy with their personal lives, compared with only 3 percent two decades earlier. Unhappiness with work jumped to 20 percent from 11 percent, and unhappiness with the community climbed to 24 percent from 13 percent. The questioners also found a sharp increase among the young of insomnia, nervousness, headaches, loss of appetite, and upset stomach—all symptoms of stress.

Item: A study of air traffic controllers, whose jobs involved long hours of anxiety and tension, found an abnormally high incidence of high blood pressure and stomach ulcers.

Item: A University of Nebraska report noted an unusual number of sudden deaths, apparently from heart attacks (50 percent higher than expected), for young space-center workers at a time of the heaviest layoffs when the space program at Cape Kennedy was winding down.

All of these reports reinforce the knowledge that stress has become a part of our lives and undoubtedly is here to stay.

THE PURPOSE OF THIS BOOK

This book will focus upon occupational distress and a reaction to it known as "job burnout." As discussed in the following chapters, job burnout is a human malfunction resulting from responses to various forms of occupational distress.

Job distress can be either physically or psychologically induced. My review of the research will not discuss in any detail the many known physical distressors (sources of distress), such as extreme heat, cold, or humidity; viruses or bacterial infections; exposure to pollutants, industrial poisons, or chemicals; infrared, ultraviolet, or nuclear radiation; noise, vibration, dangerous machinery; or other external job stressors. Instead, emphasis is placed upon those factors that affect one's psyche—an area often neglected by occupational health organizations. My investigation, then, is not of external environmental discomfort but of the force killing us from inside.

It is obvious that work places were not intended to damage employees, nor are they run for that purpose. Unfortunately, though, it comes out that way for many people. In dealing with the effects of work organizations, it is very easy to fall prey to the trap of concentrating upon illness rather than health. Too often there is emphasis on the problems rather than the benefits of organizations. This volume, although focusing on occupational distress, recognizes the positive contributions and benefits of organizations. As a matter of fact, in one survey (Levinson, 1975) it was found that 80 percent of all workers claim they would continue working even if they had enough money to make earning a living unnecessary. The majority would like to keep working—but not at the same job (p. 20).

The purpose of this book is to assist educational organizations and individuals in the identification of potential areas of distress, as well as to increase public awareness of occupational stress in education. The ultimate hope is to prevent or remediate the negative effects of occupational distress upon the health and well-being of both the educator and the organization.

Organizational stress is both powerful and insidious. If unchecked and excessive, stress becomes harmful and can damage the quality of life. The issue is not the elimination of organizational stress, but the containment of its sources. Organizational stress needs to be monitored and maintained at levels that are tolerable, humane, productive, cost-effective, and contribute positively to the growth of the employee and the organization.

It is important to point out a notable limitation of most studies of job distress. These studies generally measure with self-report instruments both perceptions of the job situation and outcomes. Because of the potential response bias inherent in this method, future reports should include some additional objective measurements of the situations and outcomes. In addition, few investigations have been of a longitudinal nature designed to test the various hypotheses or to take measurements at several points in a time sequence. Additional research on the topic is needed. However, this book will serve as a comprehensive review of research data regarding definitions, symptoms, causes, remediation, and prevention of occupational distress and job burnout. It is important to point out that the research data regarding definitions, symptoms, and general causes come from both business and education. The material, although written primarily for educators, can be applied to all organizations and occupations.

COMIC RELIEF

In the course of researching the subject matter for this book, I have encountered various pieces of wisdom that provided comic relief and, at the same time, underscored some truths about the world and work. It is my hope that the reader will also enjoy these.

Murphy's Corollary: It is impossible to make anything foolproof because fools are so ingenious.

Boling's Postulate: If you're feeling good, don't worry. You'll get over it.

Jolly's Law: If the anticipated result is positive, there will always be someone eager to believe it happened as a result of his or her own pet theory.

Job's Reality: A short cut is the longest distance between two points.

Tenth Law of Communication: The inevitable result of improved and enlarged communication between different levels in a hierarchy is a vastly increased area of misunderstanding.

First Rule of Management: No manager devotes effort to proving himself wrong.

Smith's Law: The person who can smile when things go wrong has thought of someone to blame it on.

First Law of Debate: Never argue with a fool—people might not know the difference.

Boren's Laws: When in doubt, mumble. When in trouble, delegate. When in charge, ponder.

Truman's Law: There ain't no such thing as a free lunch.

Parkinson's First Law: Work expands to fill the time available for its completion.

Parkinson's Second Law: Delay is the deadliest form of denial.

Booker's Law: An ounce of application is worth a ton of abstraction.

Peter's Corollary: Work is accomplished by those workers who have not yet reached their level of incompetence.

Bureaucratic Dogma #1: Super-competence is much more objectionable than incompetence.

Bureaucratic Dogma #2: Internal consistency is more highly valued than efficient service.

Bureaucratic Dogma #3: If there is a way to delay an important decision, the good bureaucracy, public or private, will find it.

Bureaucratic Dogma #4: A bureaucratic official would rather multiply subordinates, not rivals.

Researcher's Nightmare #1: If the facts do not conform to the reader, they must be disposed of.

Researcher's Nightmare #2: After painstaking and careful analysis of a sample, you are always told that it is the wrong sample and doesn't apply to the problem you've investigated.

Researcher's Realization #1: When researching a problem, it always helps if you know the answer.

Researcher's Realization #2: Enough research will tend to support any theory.

Hoare's Law of Large Problems: Inside every large problem is a small problem struggling to get out.

Newton's Fourth Law: Almost all great discoveries or inventions are made by mistake.

Harvard's Law: Under the most rigorously controlled conditions of pressure, temperature, volume, humidity, and other variables, the organism will do as it damn well pleases.

JOB BURNOUT IN PUBLIC EDUCATION

Symptoms, Causes, and Survival Skills

CHAPTER I

Stress and Distress

The concept of stress is as old as life itself. Prehistoric humans experienced stress from fear, disease, difficult labor, or prolonged exposure to extremes of temperature. Like us, our early ancestors realized that certain bodily reactions occurred when limits were exceeded. Today we define stress as any perceived event that causes a demand upon one's mind or body. The stressor can be physical or psychological, actual or imagined.

One cannot and should not avoid stress. Many researchers have clearly found that life *is* stress. Life without stress is death or immortality. Both pleasant and unpleasant conditions cause stress. Our bodies respond to both kinds of stress—whether it be a new baby, death of a family member, a promotion, or a severe economic recession. Any of these events prepares the body for a common stress reaction: "fight or flight." An exploration of this common reaction and the importance of the individual's perception of a stressful situation cannot be overemphasized and will be discussed later in this chapter.

In ancient China, the symbol for stress included two written characters—the ones for danger and opportunity. The *danger* of stress is the possibility of bodily harm if the source goes unchecked. The *opportunity* of stress is the possibility of its motivating effect. Thus, stress can be harmful or helpful depending upon its perceived intensity and frequency. Almost all researchers agree that a certain level of stress provides incentive. Each individual has an optimal level of motivational stress—some prefer high levels, others low levels. The same level can be either stimulating or harmful, depending upon the individual's tolerance. However, each person has a finite stress limit. If our neurological wiring overloads, it short-circuits.

Stress is a familiar concept in the context of physics. The physical sciences describe how severe stress produces deformation in metals. Hooke's law states that if the strain produced by a given stress falls within the elastic limit of the metal, when the stress is removed, the metal returns to its original condition. If the strain exceeds the elastic limit, however, then damage will result. The principle of physical stress is strikingly analogous to psychological stress. Humans have a finite degree of resistance beyond which injury occurs. Individuals can tolerate appropriate levels of stress, but when distress (inappropriate or excessive levels) occurs, temporary or permanent damage is the result.

DISTRESS

The psychological and physiological effects of stress upon man have been the focus of study in the fields of psychology, psychiatry, physiology, internal medicine, sociology, anthropology, and business. Stress becomes a problem when it ceases to be a healthy stimulus, but instead creates a burden the individual cannot handle without harmful effect. Researchers call this harmful type of stress "distress."

Several researchers have found that events do not in themselves produce distress reactions. Instead, it is one's perception of events that makes them distressful. Distress, then, is any perceived threat or discomfort that alerts the person and activates psychological and physiological responses. The harmful effects of distress can be prevented or reduced by modifying the individual's environment, perception, or state of arousal. Thus, a person may not perceive a threat as distressful if he or she feels able to successfully cope with the situation.

Because the distress syndrome requires the organism to constantly adjust and readjust, it can have a destructive effect. It is important to remember that distress and its subsequent effects should be understood as relative and cumulative, rather than absolute one-time events. Dr. Walter Cannon (1932) first described the physiological reaction to distress as "fight or flight." In times of emergency, the body automatically reacts by heightened alertness, faster heartbeat, increased respiration. In ancient times this emergency reaction was necessary for survival; it prepared the organism to either fight or flee a distressful event through swift and energetic action.

Most of modern-day stress is in the form of social constraints and worries. The emergency reaction is triggered by tension or conflict of a psychological nature. Today we trip the switch by our thought processes: if we imagine ourselves in danger by worrying about things, fight or flight results. Our thoughts convince us that there is threat of impending danger.

McGrath (1970b) emphasized that distress is the result of an imbalance between demand and the organism's capacity to meet the demand. The capacity to cope varies not only with environment and social conditions, but also with heredity, training, and health.

There are many potential occupational stressors found in education. Some psychological distressors might include an unappreciative boss, lack of clear-cut goals or duties, unrealistic expectations, too much paper work, competition with colleagues, or little opportunity for input. Since distress is a perception of a demand, situations that might cause a person to become frustrated one day cause no reaction on another day. Most important is that one's reactions are based upon beliefs. Perceptions determine responses, and a person can trigger a stress reaction through accurate or inaccurate perceptions. A teacher facing involuntary transfer can often experience more negative stress from the anticipation of the event (unknown fears) than the actual stressor itself (reassignment). The "stress of stress" is often more debilitating than the actual stressor.

Distress may also result from multiple or excessive stress events of an unpleasant nature. An example of a sequence of excessive stressors upon a school principal might include: a first-grader runs away from school; an irate parent storms into the principal's office; rain starts five minutes before lunch; a student breaks a leg; a significant error is discovered in the school budget; both the superintendent and a group of teachers express disapproval of the principal's budget management.

The effects of distress can trigger a chain reaction. The principal's day has been a disaster; he or she stews about it on the way home; directs frustration and anger toward the family; and finally, after a night of little rest, begins another school day that will probably escalate the cycle. When excessive stress turns to distress, displaced reactions often occur. Displaced fight involves an attack on someone other than the person creating the stress. Usual targets for displaced energy include one's supervisor, spouse, children, or even the family dog.

Displaced flight involves such reactions as calling in sick when excess stress is anticipated; procrastinating about stressful duties; referring angry parents to the school-district office; and withdrawing from school or social activities. Displaced flight is characterized in organizations by staff turnover, excessive sick leave, unfinished projects, and over-delegation of responsibility to others.

Distress is frequently the result of frustration through experiencing phenomena such as poor communication, inadequate rest periods, limited opportunity for growth, and other unfavorable working conditions. High productivity, esprit de corps, motivation, and effective management are attained when emotional, physical, and environmental stress factors are managed to allow for optimal individual growth and productivity. Adaptation to stress is the responsibility of both employee and employer; it provides a natural protective power that prepares one to handle unfamiliar or difficult tasks. There are few job environments that do not generate some degree of fear, overload, pressure, or frustration. When events tax an individual beyond the point of tolerance, then hypertension, lower back pain, or other identified distress maladies occur.

MAJOR RESEARCH ON STRESS AND DISTRESS

The cost of distress is enormous. Dr. Harold Bloomfield (1975) reported the following statistics:

- Five billion doses of tranquilizers, three billion doses of amphetamines, and five billion doses of barbiturates are administered through prescription each year. The great majority are for fatigue, hypertension, nervousness, and insomnia.
- Half of all deaths are linked to vascular/heart disease.
- Ten percent of American adults suffer from peptic ulcers.
- Physicians are reporting ever-increasing rates of psychosomatic illness related to stress.
- The number one health problem in the U.S. today is distress.

Two individuals, Dr. Edmund Jacobson and Dr. Hans Selye, have gained international reputations for decades in their study of stress, distress, and relaxation.

Jacobson's Research

Dr. Edmund Jacobson, an internist, diagnostician, and psychiatrist, can aptly be described as the "father of nervous tension research." He began his studies in 1908 and, although he is about ninety, continues to lecture, write, conduct research, and commute regularly between Chicago and New York. Dr. Jacobson has written 12 books and published some 73 articles.

Dr. Jacobson prefers to use the term "muscle tension" rather than stress or distress. He defines tension as the excessive contracting of muscle fibers. This tension or energy is expended in demanding situations. Relaxation is defined as the direct opposite of excessive muscle tension or the absence of unnecessary muscle contraction. According to his research, tension disorders such as peptic ulcers, spastic colon, high blood pressure, or premature heart attacks are considered the result of muscle tension.

Dr. Jacobson believes we live in a tense world. It is a subject we talk and read about regularly. Doctors and friends tell us to "relax"; however, this has not always been the case. Dr. Jacobson recalls a book on the subject of rest written during Woodrow Wilson's presidency; the word "relaxation" did not appear in the index. People at that time did not discuss tension. The characters in movies written in that epoch did not tell each other to "relax" as they do today, because the concept of stress had not yet become part of the mores of that time. Yet, ten years previously, Dr. Jacobson had already begun to study the principles of tension and relaxation as we know them now. His data suggested that in an advancing competitive society, tension disorders become more common. During difficult times, including inflation and loss of jobs, tension reduces personal efficiency.

Since 1908, members of every common profession and business have come to Dr. Jacobson's clinic with characteristic tension complaints. He has treated doctors, dentists, lawyers, engineers, executives, teachers, journalists, bankers, and publishers. During the printing of his first book, *Progressive Relaxation,* in 1929, the printers and workers at the University of Chicago Press claimed that excessive tension applied particularly to them. In later years, when he had the occasion to meet with union members of the garment and other trades, it became evident that they likewise showed marked symptoms of high tension. The same held true for other workers, and for managers, as well.

Dr. Jacobson suggests that although not scientifically proven, there is strong evidence that tension disorders are more prevalent than the common cold. Colds may last but eight days in otherwise healthy people, and recur no more than about twice a year. Tension disorders remain with us year-round. The predominance of tension disorders is validated by statistics that tranquilizers are the most common of medicines. If we add the great tranquilizer known as alcohol, the cost to relieve tension becomes staggering.

The evidence indicates that one's susceptibility to tension disorders varies with heredity as well as with environment. For example, in reviewing coronary heart disease, we cannot rule out the influence of heredity. In the male, the lining of the coronary vessels is much thicker at birth than in the female, in whom the incidence of coronary heart disease is much lower. Heart attacks generally arise from coronary sclerosis aggravated by tension. The greater the tension or the more advanced the sclerosis, the more likely the individual will suffer from coronary heart disease.

Dr. Jacobson in his famous book *You Must Relax*, first published in 1934 and now in its fifth revised edition (1978), offers an interesting anecdote on coronary disease and its relationship to tension.*

> My neighbor Harry is in the hospital. They say he has had a heart attack! Harry perhaps, is a businessman well liked by those who know him well. However, Harry could as well be disliked and he could be a factory worker, a lawyer, a doctor, an engineer, an admiral or any other type. Possibly he is forty-five or fifty years old or somewhat older, but he might be only thirty-five. There are many Harrys of many ages and this is one reason why I have written this book.
>
> What has tension to do with Harry's heart attack? Let us first consider the case for the negative—namely, that tension has little or nothing to do with bringing it on. Many people, including some doctors and even some heart specialists, still believe this. Currently among these are some who assert that whether Harry has a heart attack or not depends on the state of his coronary arteries, whether these are hardened, sclerotic. Fat, they argue, is deposited in the heart arteries, weakening their walls, thus allowing them to burst or to develop stasis within, so that blood flow to some part of the heart-wall ceases, which is what people know as a heart attack. Arteriosclerosis, they add, is the cause of coronary heart disease and tension plays only a minor role if any. At most, it aggravates the symptoms, these polemicists claim, or sets off an attack through an emotional crisis, which would have come a little later on anyway.
>
> Their arguments appear so sound, so scientific, so authoritative that we pause to wonder if they are not wholly right. Without doubt, fatty deposits are found in diseased coronary arteries. What, then, has tension to do with heart attacks? What, indeed?
>
> There was a time when our boys were dying during the war in Korea. Three hundred of them died in combat whose hearts were carefully examined subsequently. Autopsies were performed by Major William F. Enos and his associates. Even though their age averaged in the early twenties, 77 percent had some degree of disease of the coronary arteries. In many instances, the hearts were so severely diseased that the examiners were amazed. They could not understand how these hearts had held out during the battle until the boy was killed by shot and shell or other external violence.
>
> I do not know of any reasonable way to interpret the findings of

---

* From the book *You Must Relax* by Dr. Edmund Jacobson. © 1978 (5th edition), McGraw-Hill Book Company. Used with permission.

Major Enos on these poor boys of ours but that the strain and tension of the war had proved too much for their arteries. Was it their diet? Did their hearts degenerate because they ate too much fat, too much cholesterol?

No record was found and published that could support the view that they had partaken of too much cholesterol. The army diet does not provide any excess of fat. Nobody claims that it does. The fat content of meals provided for our army forces was, we can assume, approximately of the same percentage as was provided for these boys in typical American homes in peace time. So far as fat content was concerned, these boys had been eating as all Americans eat on the average.

Yet the incidence of severe coronary heart disease in these young boys was very much in excess of the incidence in American boys of the same age who had not participated in the strains and tensions of active warfare. It is said that approximately one out of two American males shows beginning hardening of the coronary arteries at the age of thirty-five or forty. But what is found in these early-middle-aged men is only the beginnings of disease, not advanced disease such as Major Enos found in many of our three hundred boys. And he found marked coronary heart disease not merely in one out of two but in the majority— namely, in about 77 percent.

The debaters therefore would find it hard to make out a case to prove that the coronary heart disease found in these fighters post mortem was due chiefly to fatty diet.

Major Enos concludes that the combatants suffered from *wear* and *tear* on the lining membranes of the coronary arteries and from *stress* at branching points. While he does not discuss the tense life at war as leading to the wear and tear and stress, his results contrast greatly with what we know of the normal, healthy hearts on the average in American boys in civilian life who have undergone no such strains. It seems safe to assume that their occupation as combatants with its extreme tensions of emotion and effort was largely responsible. (pp. 32–37)

Dr. Jacobson firmly believes that by avoiding undue tension and by the use of relaxation, we can prevent, or at least slow down the development of, tension disorders and degenerative diseases such as coronary heart disease.

Selye's Research

Beginning in 1926, Hans Selye, M.D., studied the body's physiological response to stress. Dr. Selye is now a professor and a director of medicine and surgery at the University of Montreal. He has written more than 1,400 articles and 33 books, including *The Stress of Life* and *Stress Without Distress*.

In a 1977 article,* Dr. Selye wrote:

> We can no longer count on "having finished our training" for our work
> or on "having arrived at our goal" in society; nowadays the skills and
> knowledge demanded by any job, as indeed the goals of society itself,
> are developing (or at least changing) at such an unprecedented rate
> that our first objective must be to learn how to cope with the stress of
> adaptation to change as such, both in our work and in our social goals.
> Only then can we hope to succeed in over-coming the distressing loss
> of stability and perhaps even to enjoy the challenge of adjustment to
> ever-changing tasks, aspirations, and possibilities. (p. 6)

Everyone is exposed to stress, yet the phenomenon is poorly understood by the general public. Stress is glibly discussed in social circles,
but few have bothered to define it. Many air their views about stress
in marriage, business management, or politics, yet never take time to
study the medical implications of stress.

In 1926 Dr. Selye began to wonder why patients suffering from diverse diseases had so many symptoms in common. Whether a man
suffered from severe loss of blood, infectious disease, or advanced can-
cer, he lost appetite, muscular strength, and also ambition. Usually the
patient lost weight, and even his facial expression often betrayed that
he was ill. These were the medical symptoms of what Selye called at
the time the "syndrome of just being sick."

In 1936, while seeking a new ovarian hormone, Selye injected ex-
tracts of cattle ovaries into rats to see if their organs would display
changes that could not be attributed to any previously identified hormone. Three types of reactions were noted: (1) the cortex (outer layer)
of the adrenal glands became enlarged and hyperactive; (2) the thy-
mus, spleen, lymph nodes, and all other lymphatic structures shrank;
and (3) deep, bleeding ulcers appeared in the stomach and upper intestines.

Dr. Selye soon discovered that all toxic substances, irrespective of
their source, produced the same pattern of response in the rats. More-
over, identical organ changes were evoked by cold, heat, infection,
trauma, hemorrhage, nervous irritation, and many other stimuli. Gradu-

---

* Hans Selye, "Stress Without Distress," *School Guidance Worker,* May 1977,
quoted with the permission of the Guidance Centre, Faculty of Education, Uni-
versity of Toronto, Toronto, Ontario. Material (as it appeared in *School Guidance
Worker*) abridged and adapted from Chapter Five in *Stress Without Distress* by
Hans Selye (J. B. Lippincott Company). Copyright © 1974 by Hans Selye, M.D.
Reprinted by permission of Harper & Row, Publishers, Inc.

ally, he realized that the effect of the injections in rats was an experimental replica of the human "syndrome of just being sick." Adrenal enlargement, gastrointestinal ulcers, and thymicolymphatic shrinkage were constant and invariable signs of damage to the body when it was faced with the demand of meeting an attack from any disease. These changes became recognized as objective indices of stress and furnished a basis for developing the entire stress concept.

Hans Selye (1977, p. 7) defines stress as "the nonspecific response of the body to any demand made upon it." Most drugs exert specific actions: insulin reduces blood sugar, while diuretics enhance the production of urine. Yet both produce a common reaction in the body: an overall, nonspecific response which causes the need for bodily readjustment.

Dr. Selye feels it has taken physicians a long time to accept the existence of a stereotyped body response to any kind of demand. For years it did not seem logical that different demands should cause the same response. Yet, there are many analogies in everyday life. For example, our houses have ovens, refrigerators, and light bulbs which respectively produce heat, cold, and light in a specific manner. However, the production of these forms of energy depends upon a single common factor—electricity.

It is immaterial whether a stressor is pleasant or unpleasant; all that counts is the intensity of the demand for bodily readjustment or adaptation. The mother who is suddenly told that her only son died in Vietnam suffers a terrible shock. However, if years later her son is found alive and well, she experiences extreme joy. The specific emotions resulting from the two events, sorrow and joy, are direct opposites; but their stressor effect, or nonspecific demand to readjust, is the same.

Selye does not feel that defining stress is sufficient. It is important to indicate what stress is *not*, thus dispelling misconceptions. Stress is not simply nervous tension, because stress reactions have been found to occur in lower animals or plants that do not have nervous systems. Stress is not just nervous exhaustion or intense emotional arousal. It can be the lack of emotional stimuli often observed during isolation or social ostracism.

As mentioned earlier, a stress agent can be pleasant or unpleasant. The stressor effect depends merely on the intensity of the demand made upon the adaptive capacity of the body. Indeed, stress does not have to result in any form of injury. Dr. Selye says that a game of tennis or a passionate kiss can produce considerable stress without causing damage.

Using Selye's definition, stress cannot be avoided. Even while asleep and fully relaxed a person is under some stress. That is, the heart must continue to pump blood, intestines continue to digest food, muscles move the chest to permit respiration, and the brain engages in dreams. Complete freedom from stress is death.

Dr. Selye feels that the word "stress" is often misused. In social situations, when a person says he or she is under stress, what is actually meant is excessive stress or distress, just as the statement "running a temperature" refers to an abnormally high temperature. Psychological distress often results from prolonged or unvaried stress or from frustration.

Dr. Selye has shown that animals exposed to continuous stress for long periods go through the three phases of the "General Adaptation Syndrome": initial alarm reaction, followed by resistance, and eventually exhaustion. In the same way that a machine gradually wears out, so will the human body eventually become the victim of wear and tear. Selye's research concluded that adaptability (adaptation energy) is finite. He compared it to an inherited pool of capital from which one could withdraw throughout life, but to which one could never add.

> The secret of success is not to avoid stress and thereby endure an uneventful, boring life, for then our wealth would do us no good, but to learn to use our capital wisely, to get maximal satisfaction at the lowest price. Often, the satisfaction of any experience must be bought at the price of sacrificing another. It pays to learn how not to squander this valuable asset on futilities. (1977, p. 11)

Paradoxically, the greatest experts in the field do not know why the stress of frustration rather than that of excessive muscular work is much more likely to produce disease—peptic ulcers, migraine, or high blood pressure. Physical exercise can even provide relaxation and help the person withstand mental frustration. In fact, a voluntary change of activity is even better than rest when task completion becomes stymied. Dr. Selye says that "when either fatigue or enforced interruptions prevent us from finishing a mathematical problem, it is better to go for a swim than to just sit" (1977, p. 11).

Dr. Selye concluded his treatise with the wise observation that some form of release is a biological necessity.

> Each person must find a way to relieve his pent-up energy without creating conflicts with his fellowmen. Such an approach not only ensures peace of mind but also earns the goodwill, respect, and even love of our fellowmen, the highest degree of security, and most noble "status symbol" to which man can aspire. (p. 12)

OCCUPATIONAL STRESS AND DISTRESS

The Organizational Worker

Work usually occupies the largest investment of time and energy in a person's life. Approximately 65 to 70 percent of an individual's waking hours, five days a week, is devoted to work-related activities (assuming a 40-hour week, travel time, and preparation). Most people want to do an excellent job; few, if any, actually intend to do a poor job. Employees want to do well in their occupations in order to gain a useful, productive, identity. Work can offer a major source of personal satisfaction, which may overflow into non-work life. Friendships and leisure activities are often initiated at the work place.

Many significant changes have occurred within the world of work. A century ago the 40-hour work week was not the norm, although the basic necessity to earn a living was the same as today. Our ancestors of the 1880s had no cars and little access to public transportation. They were not apt to be employed at a distant factory or office. Most of them were likely to be agrarian or crafts workers whose jobs were closely tied to their basic needs—obtaining food and shelter.

Albrecht (1979) indicated that within the past century, "the organization" has taken over our culture. Management approaches such as bureaucracy, "Theory X," or Taylorism have dominated the organizing of employees. During the 1930s, the classic management style was shattered by the Hawthorne studies.* A discovery was made which indicated that paying attention to employee needs and showing interest in employees as people greatly increased productivity. These gains in productivity far surpassed the increases achieved from technical adjustments (e.g., improvements in machines) that were also measured as part of the studies. Since that time, the importance of human relations in organizations has been emphasized by McGregor (1960), Herzberg (1959), and Likert (1961), who pointed toward more humanitarian goals as the major means of creating additional worker comfort and productivity. In the meantime, work has become progressively more technical and specialized. This inevitable progression in technology has created heretofore unimaginable products, as well as creating in workers new sources of stress that had not been anticipated.

---

* Theory X, Taylorism, and the Hawthorne studies are mentioned in most of the research literature discussed in this paragraph. They are more extensively covered in Herzberg (1959).

Bennis (1966) strongly suggests that traditional management models are no longer capable of dealing with current change. He indicates that current change is proceeding at a geometric rate such that today we view more change in a single year than our grandparents saw in a lifetime. Bennis and others have suggested that work has altered so rapidly that some organizations are unable to adapt. The bureaucratic model, for example, fails miserably in a complex, high-technology work environment. Bureaucratic models were designed to avoid change, insure stability, and provide a chain of command. This was intended to ensure speed, efficiency, continuity, and uniformity and to effectively deal with large numbers of people in fixed job categories. However, in today's highly specialized and changing world, bureaucracy is often an anachronism.

Our world is now a complex network of organizations. The organizational phenomenon is not only linked to business or manufacturing; it has spread to every segment of society, including schools, government, churches, hospitals, non-profit groups, and services ad infinitum. In order to carry out daily life, each of us must identify or align with some form of organization, whether it be large or small, democratic or autocratic. People are still striving to adapt to this immensely complicated new world. We have not learned how to deal effectively with all of the stresses that exist in the organizational environment. We are in a new era of adaptation, and the art of management remains in its infancy.

Definitions of Occupational Stress and Distress

Dr. Herbert Benson of the Harvard Medical School has pioneered studies of the effects of occupational stress on businessmen. His work is strikingly similar to that of Dr. Hans Selye. Benson equates man's nervous system to that of other animals. When an animal perceives a threat, its physiological response prepares it for flight or battle. This response, like man's, is characterized by increased metabolism, higher blood pressure, faster heart rate and breathing, and tenseness of skeletal muscles. Stress reactions, if continually stimulated, affect the body by maintaining a condition of perpetual stress. If stress is sustained, it inevitably becomes distress.

In reviewing the various conceptions of stress, McLean (1974) concluded that stress is neither stimulus, response, nor intervening variable. It is, rather, a collective term for an area of study—one which, in its broadest sense, is differentiated from other problem areas in that it deals with any demands that tax the system, whether the system be physiological, social, or psychological, and the responses of that system to the taxing demands. Job stress can result from any work situation where job-related factors disrupt or enhance a worker's physical or mental condition. McLean, however, defines an occupational (dis)-tressor* as any work-related factor which produces a maladaptive response. Occupational stress can be broadly defined as the by-product of an interaction between workers and their work environment. Occupational distress can be defined as a job-related demand that exceeds the worker's capacity.

Other researchers (e.g., McGrath, 1970a,b) have defined occupational distress as occurring when there is a substantial imbalance between environmental demands and the response capability of the employee. The individual's appraisal and anticipation of the threat of stress are equally as important as the actual demand. Distress happens if an imbalance between perceived demand and perceived ability to respond exists. When environmental work stressors are such that people can ignore them or fulfill them without serious consequences to themselves, those stressors will not generate a threat. However, if the individual perceives a demand as exceeding his or her response capability, it becomes a distressor.

It is clear, then, that the job stress phenomenon involves complicated interactions between individual and work environment. It is also evident, after consideration, that time plays an important role. For example, although an employee's job may cause stress, his or her reaction to that stress may occur immediately, later at home, or at any time in the future.

Occupational Distressors

Occupational distressors have been categorized by Albrecht (1979) as falling into four general categories:

Time Distress: A reaction to time, including the feeling that one must do something before a deadline. It also includes the distressed feeling that time is running out and something terrible may result.

Anticipatory Distress: A reaction commonly known as anticipation or worry—feeling anxious about an impending event. Often this includes a diffuse feeling of dread or the fear that something catastrophic might occur.

Situational Distress: A reaction to finding oneself in a threatening situation beyond one's control or coping ability. It may involve dan-

---

* Prefix added by author.

ger of physical injury, failure, loss of status, or lack of acceptance.

Encounter Distress: A reaction to dealing with others whom one perceives to be unpleasant or unpredictable. This apprehension is often felt by those unable to understand conventional social rules or acceptable behavior (pp. 86–87).

The Effects of Occupational Distress

In the United States more than 23 million individuals are afflicted with hypertension, 90 percent of which cannot be traced to physiological irregularities. Sixty to 80 percent of the typical doctor's caseload is reported to be directly related to distressors. Signs of job distress include high job turnover, tardiness, absenteeism, increased discontent, and slowed output. Distress accounts for more lost work time than all other causes put together. (Chapter II of this book will focus on understanding the symptoms, causes, and effects of distress.)

In the past 15 years there has been a 22 percent rise in the amount of absence from work that can be attributed to physical disease. During this same period, there has been a 152 percent increase in mental disorders among men and a concurrent increase of 302 percent among women (Kearns, 1973; National Association for Mental Health, 1971). Only one out of six workers in the labor force of the United States reports being free of tension on the job (Kahn et al., 1964). Whether the increase is due solely to occupational distress is a moot point. Sufficient evidence, however, warrants serious inquiry into the effects of distress at work.

Margolis, Kroes, and Quinn (1974a,b) define occupational distress as a condition at work interacting with worker characteristics to disrupt psychological or physiological homeostasis. These researchers define the causal conditions as job stressors, and the disrupted homeostasis as job-related strain. Margolis and colleagues suggested that there are at least five dimensions of job-related strain: short-term, subjective states (anxiety, tension, and anger); longer-term and more chronic psychological responses (depression, general malaise, and alienation); transient physiological changes (levels of catecholamine, blood pressure); physical health (gastrointestinal disorders, coronary heart disease, asthmatic attacks); and work performance decrement.

Cobb and Rose (1973) compared air traffic controllers (reported to be the highest occupational distress job) to air force personnel with respect to the incidence of two stress diseases. The prevalence of hypertension among air traffic controllers was four times higher than for the air force personnel. Also, the onset of the illness was on the average seven years sooner. Similar findings were obtained regarding peptic ulcers; the incidence was two times higher for air traffic controllers.

According to Truch (1980) teachers are becoming an endangered species. One-third of the teachers contacted in a survey said they would not go back to teaching if they had the choice to do it again. Truch reported that more medical insurance claims are being made by teachers than by members of any other profession. In England, the rate of death of male teachers near the age of retirement has doubled in ten years. Another study reported by Dr. Truch indicated that the life expectancy of a teacher is four years lower than the national life-expectancy average. Wilson (1979) found that 77 percent of the teachers surveyed reported that physical signs of distress were present much of the time. Ninety percent indicated that distress was often a cause of sick leave.

A review of health records of more than 22,000 workers in 130 occupations was conducted over a two and one-half year span (Colligan et al., 1977). The highest incidence of stress-related disease occurred among laborers, secretaries, inspectors, clinical lab technicians, and office managers/administrators. Administrators ranked in the top four of the 130 occupations for highest rates of death and hospital admission. In another study (Gmelch, 1977), it was found that two-thirds of the school administrators who responded felt that 70 percent of their total life stress was job-related.

SUMMARY

A life without stress is neither possible nor desirable. Stress at reasonable levels primes one for peak performance at work or at play. At unreasonable levels, stress becomes distress and leads to depression, illness, or apathy. It may even pave the way toward breakdown of internal organs or body systems already weakened by heredity or disease. In most people distress symptoms disappear as the causes of distress abate. For others distress becomes a chronic way of life. It has been noted that tension disorders—peptic ulcers, hypertension, and diabetes—occur more frequently among air traffic controllers, office managers, and helping professionals including school teachers and administrators than in less draining occupations. Distress can aggravate asthma, create skin rashes, bring on migraine headaches, produce ulcerative colitis, insomnia, loss of appetite, or a whole list of other symptoms.

Stress reactions are the body's natural response to a perceived challenge, causing the fight or flight syndrome. We carry with us a nervous system no different from that of our early ancestors. Then as now, at the threat of danger, blood pressure increases, muscles tense, adrenaline is pumped into the blood, heartbeat increases, eyes dilate, blood sugar increases, breathing accelerates, and blood is pumped to the brain. All of these physiological responses gear us toward action with one objective—survival.

Unfortunately, the threat to an individual need not be real; it can be imagined. It can be pleasant or unpleasant, certain or uncertain, anticipatory or after the fact. Continued excessive stress, if uncontrolled, leads to a persistent body reaction. People who experience long-term distress have bodies that are perpetually tense, inordinate levels of hormones in the blood, high blood pressure, increased digestive acids, and faster breathing, all of which are consuming unnecessary amounts of energy resulting in increased wear and tear on their bodies. We must learn to conserve our body energy by recognizing the circumstances that create undue stress. If we learn to manage harmful stressors, we can enhance our enjoyment and extend our lives.

According to Dr. Selye, each person possesses a fixed amount of adaptive energy. It is like the world's supply of oil—once depleted, it cannot be replenished. As people expend their adaptive energy in wasteful amounts, the signs of aging and fatigue become apparent. Remember that stress is cumulative. Each stress we are unable to cope with becomes distress, which, when accumulated, becomes destructive to our minds and bodies. Everyone has a physiological weakness, whether it be in one's heart, stomach, kidneys, liver, pancreas (diabetes), back, or head (migraine headaches). When distress becomes apparent, the weak link begins to break down. Unfortunately, distress in the twentieth century is here to stay. Physicians and hospitals cannot cure it. The only available solution is to understand the phenomenon, learn how to prevent it, and conserve adaptive energy by gaining control over distress.

A wise father (mine) once instructed his son that two things in work life are the keys to success and good health. He said, "The first is, don't let trivia bother you." He paused, and then added, "The second is, almost everything is trivia."

CHAPTER II

Job Burnout:
Definitions and Symptoms

Job burnout is both an occupational hazard and a phenomenon induced by distress. It is generally characterized by: (1) some degree of physical and emotional exhaustion; (2) socially dysfunctional behavior, particularly a distancing and insulation from individuals with whom one is working; (3) psychological impairment—especially strong, negative feelings towards the self; and (4) organizational inefficiency through decreased output and poor morale. Burnout has been equated by Ann Landers with acid—they both have the potential to destroy not only the container in which they are stored, but also that with which they come into contact.

The topic of job burnout has in the past few years received national attention. The phenomenon has been discussed in every major media form. A *San Francisco Chronicle* article by Joan Chatfield-Taylor (1979) described burnout as "more than the blahs." She pointed out that burnout can be a profound and lasting dread of going to work. It can mean mental and physical depletion ranging from fatigue to a full-fledged nervous breakdown. It does not occur overnight; instead, it is a cumulative process beginning with warning signals, and eventually leading to destroyed work motivation.

According to Dr. Edward Stambaugh, a practicing clinical psychologist who specializes in treating job burnout victims, as many as 10 percent of Americans succumb to the effects of burnout every year. He notes that some people are especially prone to burnout. Overcommitted individuals who approach problems enthusiastically may appear immune, yet often fall prey to burnout. Colleagues are likely to see burnout victims as competent, conscientious, creative, caring, and hardworking. Unfortunately these qualities also characterize those who cannot say no, and thus take on more than they can handle. In addition, the most difficult jobs are usually directed to these most capable, yet vulnerable, persons (Sommers, 1980).

Individuals whose jobs keep them in constant contact with other people are prime candidates for burnout, as are those whose occupations require them to make frequent life-and-death decisions. On the other hand, dentists burn out because they often deal with pain, and housewives from monotony; both are seldom thanked for their efforts. Depression due to lack of adequate job preparation, constant frustration, and high ambition matched to probable job dead ends are all contributing factors. Burnout comes from too little autonomy and a perceived lack of authority in decision making, as well as from too much work and stress. A 1977 study of Chicago teachers (Chatfield-Taylor, 1979) suggested that it was not only the constant responsibility for children and pressure from their parents that drove numbers of teachers out of the field; it was also lack of involvement in decision making, along with overcrowded classrooms and lack of materials, that caused the turnover.

DEFINITIONS OF JOB BURNOUT

A sizeable amount of research on burnout focuses primarily in two arenas: (1) helping professions, such as counselors, teachers, social workers, school administrators, psychologists, and (2) public employees, such as police, air traffic controllers, appointed officials, public health workers, and others.

Several researchers have made major contributions to the study of professional job burnout. Some of these include Herbert Freudenberger of Covenant House in New York City; Christina Maslach and Ayala Pines from the University of California, Berkeley; Leroy Spaniol and Jennifer Caputo of Human Services Associates, Lexington, Massachusetts; and Martha Mattingly of the University of Pittsburgh. Each defines and describes job burnout in a slightly different way. Following are summaries of their findings.

Freudenberger's Research

Herbert Freudenberger originally coined the term "burnout" to refer to people in the helping professions who wear themselves out in pursuit of an impossible goal. Dr. Freudenberger feels professional and public officials are constantly called upon to react unemotionally to emotional issues, particularly if the individual must maintain a public image. This work often demands that the helping professional take the role model of a selfless person expected to solve crises on a regular basis of intervention. These workers continually give emotional support, yet attempting to be non-judgmental, try to balance the contradictory values and philosophies of clients. They are besieged by "give me," "tell me," and "help me" requests. Their decisions with clients are frequently made on an immediate-demand basis that can have survival consequences for the client. It becomes progressively more difficult to leave the job at the office, because the pressure of the job follows the worker home. These constant stressors create repeated fight or flight reactions that drain the workers' energies and affect their personal lives.

Dr. Freudenberger describes the effects of burnout in these workers as cynicism, negativism, and a tendency to be inflexible and almost rigid in thinking. These characteristics often lead to a closed mind about change and innovation. Professional workers under these conditions discuss clients in intellectual terms that provide "psychological distance" as well as insulation. A subtle form of paranoia may also set in, causing the worker to feel that peers or administrators are out to make life more difficult. Another characteristic of burnout is a condescending, "know-it-all" attitude that impedes communication and creates social isolation. Paradoxically, the opposite—limited work and excessive socializing—may also occur. Some workers experiencing burnout speak of being bored and unhappy with their lot in life. They verbalize a sense of helplessness and hopelessness about themselves and their clients. They express a feeling that their work has become dull, routine, and filled with "clutter." Absenteeism, psychosomatic complaints, and real illness increase in direct relationship to the level of burnout. Unfortunately, the symptoms affect not only functioning with fellow workers and clients, but also life outside the work place. Their home lives frequently begin to deteriorate, and threats of divorce become more common.

Maslach and Pines's Research

Christina Maslach and Ayala Pines (1977) defined burnout as the "loss of concern for the people with whom one is working." In addition to physical exhaustion and illness, burnout is characterized by emotional fatigue in which the professional no longer has positive feelings, sympathy, or respect for clients or patients. A cynical and dehumanized perception of these people often develops, in which they are labeled in derogatory ways. Maslach (1976) wrote, "Our findings to date show that all of these professional groups tend to cope with stress by a form of distancing that not only hurts themselves but is damaging to all of us as their human clients" (p. 16). This affective displacement promotes the attitude that clients somehow deserve any problems they have. Consequently, as burnout increases it plays a major role in the professional's delivering poor-quality services to the people who need them most.

Failure to cope can be manifested in a number of ways. For example, burnout appears to be a factor in low worker morale, impaired performance, absenteeism, and high job turnover. A common response to burnout is to "quit and get out." Each profession refers to its own form of burnout with a different label. For example, in law enforcement it is referred to as the "John Wayne syndrome," while in teaching it is called the "rigid old lady" phenomenon. As burnout increases, so do jargon and labels (for example, "she's a classic schizo" or "he's a coronary"). Less empathy is observed as burnout becomes more severe. In its place workers develop mechanical, bureaucratic, physically distant behavior. When workers are forced to provide care for too many people, it becomes commonplace to hear comments such as "I'm sorry I can't help you, those are the rules," and "We tried that once, it didn't work."

Individuals experiencing burnout often increase their use or abuse of alcohol and tension-reducing drugs. They report the following symptoms: more mental health problems; feeling "bad, cold, calloused"; the desire to get away from people; and increased marital and family conflict. Maslach has uncovered dehumanizing response patterns which she categorized as individual detachment techniques and situational factors (to be discussed under "Dehumanization" later in this chapter).

Mattingly's Research

Martha Mattingly (1977) of the Department of Child Development at the University of Pittsburgh has also reviewed burnout as it applies to the professional child care worker. She has found an inherent and stress-producing conflict between the professional's requirement to give and the reality that he or she can never give enough. The child care professional serves children whose needs are much greater than the worker's resources can satisfy. The refreshment provided by sources such as family, friends, and colleagues was not usually found sufficient to revitalize the depleted worker.

All workers need to view themselves as successful. The experiences of success in child care work are frequently random and inconsistent. In most instances, the professional does not have the opportunity to remain involved with a child to a point of satisfactory closure.

Mattingly indicated that job descriptions are often ambiguous; many role conflicts develop not previously anticipated by child care workers or parents. Even more important is that the worker must sustain his or her professional identity with very limited reinforcement from supervisorial, social, or community contacts. This frequently results in the worker undergoing "role overload" and the community lacking understanding of the extensiveness of the job. In addition the child care worker must process an enormous amount of information at great speed, while maintaining disciplined vigilance regarding the children and the setting. Children's verbal and nonverbal behavior, changes in environment and programs, child history, and current objectives for each child are constantly registering in the worker's awareness. All of these variables interact and form the basis for hundreds of decisions the child care worker must make each day.

The child care professional works in the proverbial pressure cooker, with an extreme of interaction being an integral part of his or her daily job. The results of compressed decision making are constantly on display to the view of superiors, colleagues, and children. As Mattingly says, "The child care worker cannot turn off his tape recorder or videotape equipment or close his office door. He has few places to hide his mistakes, miscalculations, and poor decisions" (p. 129).

Spaniol and Caputo's Research

Researchers Leroy Spaniol and Jennifer Caputo (1979) defined burnout as the "inability to cope adequately with the stresses of our work or personal lives" (p. 2). They further noted,

> We can burn ourselves out when what we bring to a situation is not equal to the demands of the situation. Burnout results from the interaction between the resources we bring into a situation and the stress factors in that situation. If the stresses of our job are unusually high, the job is likely to burn us out. (pp. 2–3)

They feel burnout is harmful, not only to the person to whom it occurs, but also to the recipients of services provided by the victim. Burnout severely restricts the amount of energy available to both personal and work lives.

Spaniol and Caputo indicate that burnout reduces the energy available for constructive problem solving, innovation, and optimal effectiveness. People who experience job burnout have given beyond their limits. When professionals are drained by work conditions—particularly the needs and demands of those served—they are less able to cope successfully. The concomitant result can be less personal investment, less production, and withdrawal from social work activities.

SYMPTOMS OF JOB BURNOUT

The person who is "burning out" is usually aware only of a vague, undefined feeling of distress. These feelings are inner directed and are usually nonspecific. Burnout generally involves a reluctance to go to work, dissatisfaction with one's performance, growing fatigue, and less response in social situations. Problems at home seem to become as serious as problems at work. This painful and debilitating malady soon convinces the sufferer that he or she has less worth, less skill, and less intelligence than ever before. As the burden of distress becomes more intense, simple things such as loud noises, squabbles among children, or requests by a boss cause inappropriate or overly heightened emotional reactions. Feelings of weakness and inadequacy create a strain within work and family relationships. Introspection becomes draining and self-destructive. The worker thinks, "I must be going crazy," as others begin to ask, "What's wrong?"

Job burnout, like all distress maladies, is progressively destructive. Spaniol and Caputo have viewed the symptoms in a progression equated to varying degrees of traumatic burn injury:*

First degree: The signs and symptoms of burnout are occasional and short-lived. By providing distractions such as rest, relaxation, exercise, hobbies, or "time out," one can successfully return to a normal level of job satisfaction.

Second degree: Symptoms become more regular, last longer, and are more difficult to overcome. Normal attempts to rest and relax do not appear to be effective. After a night of sleep, the sufferer wakes up tired. Even after a weekend the victim is still tense and not ready to take on a full day's work without feeling tired. By the end of the week, the worker is exhausted and needs to dip deeply into his or

---

* Used by permission of L. Spaniol and J. Caputo, from *Professional Burn-out: A Personal Survival Kit,* © 1979, Human Services Associates.

her reserves to gain any new energy. A cynical attitude develops and is usually directed toward supervisors, supervisees, and recipients of services or products. Mood changes are noticeable. Concern over effectiveness becomes a central and disturbing issue.

Third Degree: At this level symptoms are continuous. Often, physical and psychological problems develop that are not quickly relieved with conventional medical or psychiatric attention. Self-doubt about one's competence becomes pervasive. Depression and negative feelings toward the self are rampant, with limited insight on the part of the sufferer regarding their causes. Social withdrawal from work and personal relationships becomes apparent. Serious consideration is given to finding another job or simply quitting the profession altogether. Family problems can intensify and lead to marital separations.

According to Alec Calamidas, consultant and lecturer on management development for industry and government, burnout symptoms become evident when employees begin to live only for weekends, vacations, and eventually retirement. Sayings such as "Thank God it's Friday" become symbolically commonplace in the early stages of burnout. The symptoms of progressive stages of burnout identified by Calamidas (1979a) are listed below:*

Physical Burnout Stage
  Constant fatigue.
  Noticeable physical drain.
  Minor ills become everyday ailments with lingering effects.

Intellectual Burnout Stage
  Evidence of information overload.
  Inattention; lack of concentration.
  Reduced alertness.
  "Time watching."
  Missing deadlines or doing tasks at the last minute.

Social Burnout Stage
  Irritability or being outright rude.
  Not wanting to deal with people.
  Constantly putting off necessary interactions.
  Covert desire to "play games" during interaction.
  Behavior transfer from problem area to other activities.
  Perception of not having time or desire to put off projects.

---

* Adapted by permission of Alec Calamidas.

Psycho-Emotional Burnout Stage
Conscious decision to miss deadlines.
Feeling that too much is demanded of burned out person.
Feeling that one's efforts are geared toward meeting needs of others.
Continual boredom with present, burnout environment.
Alienation and refusal to get involved with tasks involving people.

Spiritual (Dealing with Self) Stage
Needs of others become a threat.
Value system breaks down.
Little or no personal effectiveness.
No link to societal contributions.
Desire to change location or environment.
Job divorce.
Desire to escape (p. 1).

Calamidas expressed the belief that job burnout, although common to the professional who works under the bureaucratic umbrella and helping services, strikes industry in a similar manner. Most, if not all, burnout symptoms are found in industry as well as government and professional occupations. Taking his model and employing the studies by Anderson (see Askins, 1979), Collea (1979), Freudenberger (1975), Maslach (1977), Mattingly (1977), and Spaniol and Caputo (1979), a comprehensive assessment of symptoms can be developed. The following symptoms are grouped according to Calamidas' progressive stages of burnout. The reader will find them neither unusual nor surprising. In fact, it is difficult to find anyone totally free of all the symptoms.

Physical Symptoms

Fatigue/Exhaustion

The feeling of exhaustion after a draining day is common to any work. However, when burnout becomes a serious factor, exhaustion occurs on a regular basis. Fatigue is a natural sensation that reminds individuals of their vulnerability. This protective mechanism suggests the need for change or rest, which if unheeded can cause injury or collapse. Repetitive fatigue leads to chronic fatigue. Cues are needing more sleep than usual yet still lacking energy, and needing more days off. Sleep disturbances, especially insomnia, can be a consequence as well as a cause of fatigue. If not arrested, fatigue leads to such real physical ailments as ulcers, migraine headaches, or lower back pain. According to Wahlund and Nerell (1977) 48 percent of the high-stress employees in their study were too tired after work to engage in hobbies, meet friends, or perform other activities. Forty-six percent found it hard to get their minds off work.

Tenseness of Muscles and Physical Ailments

Dr. Edmund Jacobson (1978) defined tension as the tightness or contraction of muscle groups associated with stressors. In early stages neck ache, lower back pain, and/or tightness within the whole body are common complaints. Migraine headaches, stomach problems, colitis, high blood pressure, or "administrative tremor" (a shaking of the hand, voice, or body) can result. Simply put, the body is placed in a slow destructive sequence of organ burnout.

Accident Proneness

Many researchers have investigated the relationship between accidents and personal crises. When a person is under distress, accidents are more likely because one focuses less on the physical environment and ends up bumping, tripping, or falling. Schwartz (1974) even suggested that work units under high stress can be identified simply on the basis of accidents and health problems that occur within them.

Physical Distance

A relatively subtle physical symptom can be evidenced as burnout proceeds to second- and third-degree levels. Due to job pressures, individuals begin to become more physically distant from others (less touching, decreased eye contact).

High Blood Pressure

Dr. Edward J. Stainbrook, professor emeritus of psychiatry and behavioral sciences at the University of Southern California School of Medicine, observed, "In this country over the past 20 years, there has been an average increase in the diastolic blood pressure of the population . . . by several points. That indicates that there may be, as measured by this body response, just a generally increased level of tension" (Dean, 1979). Other researchers cite an epidemic of high blood pressure. More than one-third of the U.S. work force has significantly above-average blood pressure.

Use of Drugs and Alcohol

The use of drugs and alcohol can unfortunately be a means to attempt escape from stress. Drugs and alcohol may provide transient relief from tension. These artificial relaxers usually depress the central nervous system temporarily. Attempting continued stress relief by increased amounts of alcohol or drugs presents a real danger to those undergoing increased job pressure.

Heart Disease and Mental Health

A substantial amount of research has been conducted in recent years regarding occupational stress and consequent physiological and mental dysfunction. Cary Cooper and Judi Marshall (1976) of the University of Manchester Institute of Science and Technology completed a comprehensive review of the literature related to coronary heart disease and mental ill health. Their findings provide supportive evidence that "the work environment and modern organizations have an impact on the physical and mental health of their members."

Although their study is now somewhat dated, Felton and Cole in 1963 estimated that all cardiovascular diseases accounted for 12 percent of the time lost by the working population in the U.S., resulting in a total economic loss of about $4 billion in a single year. As Aldridge (1970) indicates, a report by the Department of Health and Social Security in the United Kingdom shows that the sum of incapacity for men suffering from mental, psychoneurotic, and personality disorders, nervousness, debility, and migraine headaches accounted for 22.8 million work days lost in 1968 alone (second only to bronchitis in the table of illness and lost working days). Coronary heart disease and mental ill health together, therefore, represent a serious cost for industry both in human and financial terms.

In 1975, one to three million Americans suffered some form of heart disease. Of that number, some 675,000 will die of it, 175,000 before they reach the age of 65. To most these statistics are frightening enough; however, the statistics for upwardly mobile young male and female executives and administrators are even more alarming.

In recent years Drs. Meyer Friedman and Ray Rosenman (1974), both San Francisco cardiologists, have identified a stress-prone personality type consisting of aggressive, competitive, impatient people. They have found a high rate of coronary disease among these individuals whom they call "Type A" personalities (see Appendix B). The information suggests that the individual who manifests Type A behavior may, under stress conditions, be less likely or able to control or reduce stress than the "Type B" personality. The Holmes-Rahe life-events scale measures psychological distress generated by a change in the pattern of events in a person's daily life (see Appendix A). In use since 1965, it has been found to have high validity in predicting general stress disease, especially heart attack.

Drs. Friedman and Rosenman, in their book *Type A Behavior and Your Heart,* indicate that the Type A personality suffers from "time sickness"—a feeling that there is not enough time. This causes the individual to strive to accomplish too much or to participate in too many activities in the time allotted. One characteristic of time sickness is the tendency to engage in polyphasic activity (for example, eating while reading, or driving and listening to a taped lecture). This tendency to "time bind" causes the individual to establish self-imposed deadlines, engage in rapidity of action and multiple thinking. Richard Suinn (1976) and others feel there is an inextricable relationship between distress, coronary-prone behavior, and heart attack.

The distress theory of heart attacks is certainly not new. One of the earliest accounts of a heart attack was in the Old Testament (I Samuel, 25). The emotion of anger in a rich, important man called Nabal, who was known to be "churlish and evil in his doings," finally caused his heart to die within him.

Other possible bodily warning signs of distress are:

Bruxism (teeth grinding).
Insomnia, which is usually the result of being "keyed up."
Increased activity or the inability to sit quietly or relax in a chair.
Stuttering, stammering, or increased speech difficulty.
High-pitched voice or nervous laughter.
Trembling or nervous tics.
Floating fear or anxiety without knowing its cause.
Feelings of unreality, dizziness or weakness, or orientation problems.
Dryness in the mouth or throat.
Pounding of the heart or general excitability.
Tendency to be easily startled.
Excessive sweating.
Loss of or excessive appetite.
Increased smoking.
Frequent nightmares.
Stomach or intestinal disorders.
Impeded sexual function.

Intellectual Symptoms

Impairment of Decision-Making Skills

As stressors increase to distress proportions, decision making can assume a perfunctory, delayed, or vacillating nature. Decisions either become unemotional and nonmeaningful or so difficult to make that fear overwhelms each new decision. Rational justification and enthusiasm seldom precede and follow each decision. An "I can't win" attitude begins to engulf the employee. Taking responsibility for even small decisions becomes difficult.

Deficiencies in Processing of Information

Some individuals who are quite proficient in management of details are subject to distress when faced with an overload of information which they feel obliged to analyze or otherwise process. A major characteristic of overload is the inability to focus on a single task without becoming distracted by other issues. As alertness diminishes it is followed by a typical survival response—fight or flight. Frequently the flight response becomes evident in the form of obliviousness to fellow employees, a dazed appearance, or a look of preoccupation. Fight responses such as easily provoked anger or unreasonable resentment can also be observed during overload conditions.

Time Distress

As a job becomes more aversive, a distress reaction may be the anxious anticipation of an opportunity to leave work at the earliest possible moment. The opposite reaction—becoming overwhelmed with work and ignoring the time—is equally symptomatic of distress. When either occurs, the worker may miss deadlines by procrastination or work overload. A cycle begins: reduced concentration and alertness contribute to time-related problems, while time becomes a major block to job completion.

Obsessive Thinking About Work

An unrelenting flow of thoughts about work, which occurs not only on the job but continues at home during evenings and weekends, is usually symptomatic of overinvolvement. The incapability to control work-related thoughts leads to inability to concentrate on enjoyable activities. When an employee begins to find it difficult to relax because of a stream of thoughts and concerns about work, it is a danger signal of impending burnout.

Social Symptoms

Marriage to the Job

Burnout may soon result when an employee begins to merge his or her personal life and work life. Spending many extra hours at work, taking home a large volume of work, becoming overinvolved with job-related clubs or organizations, volunteering to take on extra tasks, inviting fellow employees to share their projects or problems in off hours, working through lunch, attending weekend work-related conferences, are all examples of marriage to the job. Such overinvolvement can eventually induce distress, especially if supervisors begin to expect its regular occurrence. It is a myth to think that the work place can meet all personal needs. One must develop healthy non-work enjoyment to balance the huge amount of energy consumed in the work situation. The marriage of work and home eventually evolves into a situation most people find oppressive.

Social Withdrawal

Information overload, emotional distress, or physical debilitation may cause a person to flee from the barrage of stimulation. By avoiding contact with people, the employee may attempt to find escape from additional tension. In some cases, vulnerable individuals fear that contact with others might expose their inability to cope or verify their assumed "craziness." There is a compulsion to avoid contact in order to hide depression, anxiety, or a sense of failure.

Social withdrawal may take the form of avoiding fellow employees during lunch periods, shunning work-related social functions, or not sharing personal experiences. Pessimism pervades behavior, small talk declines, and warmth is almost nonexistent. The worker avoids walking around at the work place for fear of encountering other employees. Eye contact and nonverbal communication betray nervousness or mistrust, and anxiety in social situations becomes increasingly apparent. Mood changes are observed more frequently, communication becomes perfunctory, and positive feedback is ignored or discounted. A major personality change seems to be occurring.

As withdrawal becomes severe, communication with others in a simi-

lar plight provides little if any cathartic relief. The individual sometimes feels he or she is being rejected. Eventually, social isolation obvi-
ates any possible relief that might be offered by peers. At this point,
second- or third-degree burnout is inevitable.

Complaints/Cynicism

Distress can lead to the employee's indulging in complaints and cynicism as means to release frustration. When efforts are stymied, when
positive feedback is not forthcoming, or when a worker feels overwhelmed, the resulting anger is often vented through a hypercritical
attitude. Lashing out at fellow workers, criticizing the work environment, and being cynical in social relationships are symptomatic of impending burnout. The use of contemptuous or offensive remarks is
highly indicative of second- and third-degree burnout. It has been observed that a quick method of determining job burnout in individuals
subject to high levels of stress is to observe their behavior in the coffee
room.

Decreased Effectiveness

A worker's efficiency can be substantially affected by low morale and
job dissatisfaction. When an employee becomes this affected, deadlines
are often apt to be missed, absenteeism increases, drug or alcohol problems develop, and job output decreases in quantity and quality.
Whether it be a secretary or a teacher or a principal, just one worker's
decreased effectiveness can slowly strangle an organization. The secretary gets further behind, the teacher misses deadline after deadline, the
principal becomes less available and is less attentive to clients. The
vicious circle of poor morale, job dissatisfaction, and turnover accelerates.

Malicious Humor

Laughing with others can be a healthy release of tension. Humor
makes stress less serious and more tolerable. However, laughing at
others in a demeaning way may be a symptom of burnout. Jokes about
clients which involve a slur about their personality, culture, or social
habits may be indicative of severe emotional distress. The chronic lack
of humor and the ubiquitous presence of malicious humor are both
evidence of burnout.

Relationships at Home

If stress cannot be resolved at work, it is often more convenient to release it at home. A typical sequence finds a superintendent placing pressure upon a principal, who in turn intimidates a teacher. The teacher then extends the anger to his spouse, children, dog. When stress becomes overwhelming, it is not unusual for the ensuing frustration to be displaced upon someone innocent of involvement. A family member is frequently the target; it is easier to get angry at a spouse or child than at a boss or fellow worker. Family problems become exacerbated when stress is not resolved in the work place. High-stress occupations have historically been plagued with high rates of divorce, suicide, and family problems (administrators, police, air traffic controllers, and psychiatrists have a substantially higher incidence of these problems than the general public). It is important to view these problems as occupational consequences rather than as attributes of the worker's personality.

Aversive Associations and Social Isolation

As employee burnout reaches the third-degree level, certain job necessities become nearly intolerable. Avoidance behaviors such as telephone phobia are common. The fear of talking to or meeting with others may become obsessive. Such phobic response can lead to social withdrawal and eventually to complete isolation.

Psycho-Emotional Symptoms

Denial or Blame

A common response to major crisis or traumatic event is the denial of its existence. Frequently the immediate response to unpleasant news is disbelief. Defensive behavior and blame are close relatives to denial. Educators faced with evidence of poor performance usually deny the fact, rationalize, or blame others.

Social scientists have for years considered psychological defense as the strongest single human drive. Stronger than the desire for sex, and more urgent than the need for food or shelter, one's defenses protect the mightiest of fortresses—the ego. Loss of ego is tantamount to suicide. When stress appears likely to become continual or excessive, the organism must shore up its ego defenses. Survival, then, can mean denial, rationalization, or blame. By denying or rationalizing responsibility, the individual is protected from the pain of further insult.

Ryan (1971) found that professionals under stress have a tendency to blame clients for their problems. As pressures mount, it is tempting for the teacher to project blame onto students ("lazy, underprivileged, incorrigible") or parents ("not interested, disorganized, unwilling to cooperate"). Few attribute the cause of students' failure at school to a poor learning environment or to other factors affecting classroom effectiveness. As a result, the teacher feels less responsible for students' learning difficulties and ultimately provides less personal service.

First-degree burnout almost invariably involves a certain level of denial and rationalization. As burnout proceeds, initial defenses give way to the projection of blame. When blaming others provides little relief, self-condemnation may result. If self-blame becomes pervasive, second- and third-degree burnout soon follow.

Anger and Depression

As job pressure becomes intense, feelings of anger or melancholy can turn into full-blown episodes of depression. Anger often precedes depression, and it is interesting to note that some authors have described depression as "anger turned inward." Both anger and depression can become destructive. Anger turned outward is usually directed at those close to you (spouse, children, friends at work), alienating them and creating a vicious circle of guilt and greater stress. Anger turned inward in the form of depression also alienates others and accelerates a similar destructive cycle.

Paranoia

Trust and reliance upon others is crucial in any organization. When a worker begins to question his or her own competence, trust of others likewise becomes problematic. Fear of another taking over one's job seems real. When self-competence is questioned, competitiveness may become focused on job descriptions or other manifestations of authority. Boundaries are established and if anyone crosses those boundaries, an immediate defense is waged to maintain territorial control. Concern about the actions of others affecting one's job performance or image can become obsessional, and can result in the paranoid employee's taking malicious retribution.

Among employees in any profession, success on the job is impeded by lack of trust and the absence of cooperative interaction. Paranoid behavior results in poor worker relationships and leads to even greater distress in the employee. It has been referred to by some as a common occupational hazard among educators.

Dehumanization

For educators as well as for other helping professionals, more attention and research have been focused on the dehumanizing effects of job burnout than on any other single factor. Detachment is a natural response to overinvolvement. In order to cope with the continuous stress that results from helping others, professionals frequently reduce strain by successfully becoming detached.

Lief and Fox (1963) found that a paradox existed in the work of helping others; the paradox is that there must be a certain amount of distance (detached concern) between helping professional and client. Because there is virtually no training in such techniques, many helping professionals are unable to maintain a healthy amount of distance between themselves and clients. What frequently happens under distress conditions is a loss of concern or almost total detachment from the client that can severely dehumanize the relationship. This results in a poor quality of service.

Dehumanization literally places the client in a tightly defined category to be viewed analytically with a minimum of emotion, not unlike a laboratory specimen under microscopic examination. A large quantity of paper work is often imposed by the bureaucracy on the provider and client to justify the detachment and to continue the two-dimensional relationship between them. Regulations and policies are developed that help regulate procedures into tidy, protectively sterile, operations.

Maslach (1977) has divided the dehumanized detachment techniques into the following areas:*

> Semantics of Detachment: Terms are used to describe people more as objects and as less than human. Derogatory labels (punks, animals, or pigs), abstract or generalized terms (low SES, or medicare folk), and professional jargon (schizos, coronaries, or hypers) are all examples of how language tends to objectify people (p. 6).
>
> Intellectualization: A similar language technique reduces the situation to more intellectual and less personal terms. Abstract rather than human qualities are assigned to problem individuals. ("She displays the symptoms of behavior for a typical obsessive-compulsive type" [p. 7].)

---

* Used by permission of Christina Maslach, from "Burn-out: A Social Psychological Analysis" (paper presented at the A.P.A. Convention, August 1977). To be published in J. W. Jones (Ed.), The Burnout Syndrome (Chicago: London House Press, in press).

Situational Compartmentalization: Many educators prefer not to discuss their work. Many agencies have rules that clients not be seen, socialized with, or discussed. Consequently, little talk about the job or social contact with clients is made. Sometimes educators are embarrassed to admit their occupations. Instead they might say, "I work for the government" or "I'm in education" (p. 7).

Psychological Withdrawal: In order to stay objective and unemotional, many teachers suffering from burnout avoid even the most remote intimate interaction by keeping physical distance (avoiding eye contact, standing far away), talking in generalities, using form letters, and spending the least possible amount of time with clients. Expending time on paper work or socializing only with fellow staff members also aids in psychological withdrawal.

Unfortunately, persons who dehumanize others unknowingly rob themselves of their own humanity by creating a wall around themselves (pp. 7–8).

Self-Deprecation

Some individuals who experience work performance failure at first feel less confident, then helpless, and finally hopeless. A pervasive sense of incompetence and self-blame begins to enter private thoughts, first intermittently and then regularly. Even when one recognizes that occupational stress is a major factor, a person may still feel a sense of individual failure ("I should have been able to stand the pressure"). Unfortunately, it becomes more the rule than the exception that workers who experience burnout lay the major blame upon themselves and do not share their feelings with others. Whether from embarrassment, guilt, inability to identify causes, or social withdrawal, self-deprecating feelings fester and begin to have devastating effects upon the one afflicted.

Many employees believe their problems are self-caused, because they think their difficulties are unique and not shared by others. In regard to the helping professionals, Maslach expressed the belief that

it is easy to attribute the problem to oneself as a function of administrative response. When difficulties arise, administrators and supervisors are prone to see the problem in terms of people who are not doing their job well, rather than of short-comings in the institution itself—for which they might be implicated. It is assumed that problems are due to errors, faulty judgment, or laziness on the part of the employees, and as administrators, it is their job to improve employee performance. (p. 17)

When employees complain about organizational pressure, the pat answer is "If you can't take the heat, get out of the kitchen." This type of response reinforces self-deprecation and increases job burnout.

Self-blame results in anger, pain, or depression and causes a need to seek additional scapegoats. The educator who is burning out feels anger toward self, and soon the hostility and resentment become directed at clients. Clients are seen as deserving their problems. The professional's use of the medical model which looks for disease and ignores healthy components adds further negative focus. If the majority of an educator's time is spent with problems, it further depletes the energy of the professional. Little time is then spent on the positive attributes of clients. Success is sometimes further limited by a heavy work load or the severity of client problems. Also, as distress mounts, progress and positive feedback decrease. As apparent failure grows, so do self-deprecation and dehumanization of clients. Recipients are more likely to be perceived as incorrigible, defective, unwilling to change, hopeless, and a waste of effort. These experiences and perceptions complete a vicious circle of negativism, projection of inward ill feelings, and self-destruction.

Rigid Attitudes and Stubborn Resistance to Change

When an individual burns out, he or she becomes rigid and inflexible about procedures. Suggestions or new ideas will never work because "it costs too much"; "we tried it once"; or "you'll never convince the board" (see Appendix H). These myopic perceptions keep conditions constant and conventional. The old approach is perceived to be safe because it means less work and less stress. The worker ignores outmoded practices or new conditions and simply maintains old procedures. To maintain self-confidence, the worker thinks, "it can only work if I do it myself and ignore any changes."

Spiritual Symptoms

When burnout proceeds to its final stages, almost everything becomes a threat to the ego. Symptoms of physical distress become regular, self-confidence has reached an all-time low, and perceived work effectiveness is in a state of shambles. The worker's value to the organization is felt to be at best a token. Social relations are severely strained, and the need to change or escape is foremost in the mind of the distraught employee. The worker can perceive only the alternatives of retirement, job change, therapy, and, sadly, suicide in some cases.

As research data mount, the reality of burnout magnifies. Job burnout is very real, highly destructive, and expensive. The cost lies not only in lost production, but more importantly in lost people. Effects include:

Production Reduction

Alec Calamidas, Penn State researcher in the area of job distress, estimates that frustration robs some $500 billion from our economy (Gross National Product). He states:*

> Frustration and related stress problems cost the American economy billions of dollars each year in such areas as lost productivity, absenteeism, job turnover, vandalism/theft and illness. Distress accounts for more lost time than all other causes put together. It sets in when constant work overload, monotony and frustration overload a person mentally and physically. The most obvious signs of distress are tardiness, absenteeism, increased accident rate, diminished output, low morale and the development of escape habits such as drinking. Where frustration is deeply rooted in an organization, workers often give up serious attempts to solve problems.
>
> After frustration and related stress, job burnout is the second most important productivity and profitability killer in organizations and can affect physical, intellectual well being and social interaction. It is present in environments that include: stagnation, nonexistent delegation, unrealistic deadlines, overcontrol, insensitivity, lack of trust, no opportunity for growth and management manipulative strategies. (1979b)

Quality of Work

Given less energy, motivation, and job satisfaction, it logically follows that the quality of work will likewise decline. This can and does occur even when the quantity of work remains the same or decreases. In addition, preoccupation with trivia or lack of attention to detail can happen concurrently. Forgetting, delaying, poor attention, failing to plan—all contribute to diminished quality.

Absenteeism

In a study conducted in the United Kingdom (Aldridge, 1970), it was found that 22.8 million work days were lost in 1968 alone due to

---

* Used by permission of Alec Calamidas.

distress. There appears to be a direct relationship between level of distress and increased sick leave, lateness for work, and turnover.

Workers' Compensation Claims

Recent data on claims for workers' compensation indicate an increase of 10–15 percent in the cases settled on the basis of accumulated job stress.

Vandalism and Pilferage

Acts of vandalism and theft by employees have been described as a manifestation of tension and frustration. According to Dr. Edward Stainbrook, if tension is not discharged it is displaced, and the distressed worker reaches a point where he or she perceives the organization as so impersonal, callous, or reprehensible that stealing or sabotage is rationalized as appropriate behavior (Dean, 1979). As a consequence, more than 300,000 security guards were added by industrial firms in the United States in 1978 alone.

DISTRESS CAN BE CONQUERED

Despite dozens of studies within the past 20 years which report that people in high-distress occupations suffer a high risk of disease, succumbing to distress is not inevitable. There continue to be many people who work long hours at difficult jobs without becoming ill. Two University of Chicago researchers, Suzanne Kobasa and Salvatore Maddi (1979), have distinguished persons who manifest such characteristics as being "hardy" and more immune to disease. Their studies involve the incidence of life stress and illness among hundreds of selected occupations. The researchers have found that stress-resistant people possess a different set of attitudes about work and life. They have an openness to change, a feeling of involvement, and a sense of control over events. Basically, they perceive change as an opportunity or challenge rather than a threat, they are actively involved and committed to their work, and they take charge or control over their destiny rather than feeling powerless. Kobasa and Maddi, like Dr. Hans Selye, whose research is discussed in Chapter I, are opposed to the idea that stress should be avoided. Instead, they feel that distress can and should be mastered.

SUMMARY

Occupational distress causes varying degrees of job burnout. Although not a new phenomenon, job burnout has received a recent surge of national attention. Many researchers have undertaken the study of its symptoms and effects. There are many occupations where occupational distress is high. In addition to police and air traffic controllers, teachers and school administrators are prime victims of this destructive malady. However, there is ample evidence that occupational distress and job burnout exist to at least some degree in every occupation.

Job burnout can be defined as human malfunction resulting from various forms of occupational stress. It is manifested by a continuum of symptoms from mild to severe. Some researchers categorize burnout as progressing from minor, first-degree burns to devastating, third-degree burns; others describe the phenomenon as stages, beginning with infrequent physical ailments and graduating to severe levels of psychological and spiritual depletion. Symptoms of serious job burnout almost always include physical and emotional exhaustion, socially dysfunctional behavior, strong negative feelings toward oneself and the work place, and organizational disruption or inefficiency.

Educators and helping professionals in particular usually display some or all of these symptoms: fatigue, cynicism, negativism, apathy, rigidity, self-defeat, depression, overload, suspicion, and decreased effectiveness. As burnout symptoms replace more healthy characteristics, the educator becomes less efficient in providing services to children and parents. The increased level of burnout among educators has become a serious national problem that could eventually erode economic productivity in the business and industry sector. If educational burnout progresses to epidemic levels, its effects could cripple our economy by resulting in inadequately prepared young adults. The quality of work life is a subject that affects both private and public organizations. Certainly it is a subject that needs careful attention and consideration. Fortunately, there is both hope and evidence that occupational distress can be conquered.

CHAPTER III

Major Causes of
Occupational Distress
and Job Burnout

There is a growing body of evidence from studies in experimental laboratory settings (Kahn & Quinn, 1970) and in the work place (Margolis, Kroes, & Quinn, 1974a) to suggest that occupational distress causes health problems and job burnout. By occupational distress we mean negative environmental factors or stressors (work overload, role conflicts/ambiguity, poor working conditions) associated with a particular job. In addition to environmental factors, inherent characteristics of the individual and his or her behavior may also contribute to occupational ill health. Thus, at least two types of factors interact to determine successful coping or maladaptive behavior: (1) occupational environment, and (2) individual characteristics (personality, family, finances, or life crises). Appendix J provides a comprehensive yet nonexhaustive listing of identified stress factors adapted from Beehr and Newman (1978).

As in other maladies, the effects of job burnout vary because of individual differences. All human beings are different physically, mentally, hereditarily, experientially, and educationally. Consequently, their resistance to stress varies. Each individual has a tolerance level that is finite. At some point even the most resilient person can succumb to occupational distress.

The question of why certain people become ill and others don't under similar stressful conditions is being pursued by several research projects. The University of Chicago (Kobasa & Maddi, 1979) studied middle- and upper-level executives at a public utility whose officers were worried about the level of employee stress. Among managers who said they had experienced life crises of a degree that would ordinarily produce high levels of stress, the researchers found distinct differences between those who subsequently became ill from high blood pressure, ulcers, muscle problems, and those who remained healthy.

The "hardy" managers seemed to have a greater sense of control over their lives and a commitment to themselves. They viewed change as a challenge. In contrast, stress-susceptible managers seemed to have an aversion to change and didn't have the same sense of control over their lives. They viewed their work as competitive and pressured because of time. When faced with stressful situations, they tended to withdraw, get depressed or angry, and reduce other activities.

Some jobs, like those of symphony conductors, major league baseball players, college professors, corporate executives, and researchers, are minimally stressful, and therefore people who occupy them tend to live longer than average. Middle managers, public administrators, secretaries, and unskilled laborers experience great stress and live comparably shorter lives.

Job burnout, as mentioned earlier, is caused by the individual's inability to deal effectively with occupational distress. Researchers have identified a multitude of stressors that cause illness and job burnout. Gavin and Axelrod (1977), in a comprehensive review of 27 stressors, clearly showed that job ambiguity, role conflict, job security, participation in decision making, work load, and under-utilization of skills had demonstrable ties to psychological job distress.

THE SEVEN MAJOR CAUSES OF JOB BURNOUT

Seven causes of job burnout have received the most frequent attention in research findings.* In addition, factor analytic studies and rank order studies have shown significant relationships between these seven factors and perceived occupational stress. The seven causes are: lack of control over one's destiny; lack of occupational feedback and communication; work overload or underload; contact overload; role conflict/ambiguity; individual factors; and training deficiencies.

---

* It is important for the reader to be aware that many research citations in this book are from the literature on stress in business and industry. The major causes of stress appear to apply to many occupations.

ORGANIZATIONAL AND ENVIRONMENTAL CAUSES

Lack of Control Over One's Destiny

According to Robert Butler, Director of the National Institute on Aging (Proctor, 1979), "People who are healthy and live somewhat longer have a sense of predictability and control over their lives." Those who feel powerless and helpless tend to be less enthusiastic and give less to their work. The political nature of some jobs creates a double bind for many employees. The school principal who is wedged between conflicting federal and state laws, beset by bureaucracy, and caught between supervisorial pressure and teacher demands is caught in the bind. As organizations become large and impersonal, employees are frequently less involved in decision making. Even simple tasks can be delayed due to legal dictates, administrative policy, or lack of funds. There is massive research data outlining the effects of lack of participation in decision making. Some of the more significant studies are as follows:

- As early as 1960, Vroom reported that employee participation in decision making promotes more positive job attitudes and greater motivation for effective performance. When those persons affected by policies or decisions are involved in their creation, morale is high and stress is minimized.
- Davis and Scott (1969) found that professional personnel desire and respond favorably to a high degree of autonomy. The research team found that in an autonomous environment, the employee's morale "will be measured by his commitment to his task and his team because he will see these as instruments for his self-actualization."
- Neff (1968) summarized the importance of participation and involvement in decision making by stating, "Mental health at work is to a large extent a function of the degree to which output is under the control of the individual worker."
- Keninons and Greenhaus (1976) found that those individuals who had internal control of their work perceived more autonomy, had higher performance, and received more positive feedback than those who felt external control over their work.
- Rogers (1975) found that the two major causes of distress among administrators were work load and lack of involvement in decision making.
- French and Caplan (1970) found that people who reported more opportunities for participation in decision making reported signifi-

cantly higher job satisfaction, higher self-esteem, and low feelings of job threat.

- Buck (1972) found that managers and workers who felt under pressure viewed their supervisors as not allowing participation in decision making or consideration of new ideas.
- Margolis et al. (1974) found that nonparticipation in work decisions was the most consistent and significant predictor of job-related distress in a sample of 1,400 workers.

The findings of research data clearly indicate that greater participation in decision making results in greater productivity, higher job satisfaction, and lower employee turnover.

Lack of Occupational Feedback and Communication

Feedback. Occupational feedback is defined as the flow of job-relevant information from one employee to another. Everyone needs feedback. Infants learn to walk, talk, touch, develop tastes, through the feedback of experience and practice. Few homes are without mirrors or a bathroom scale to monitor appearance and provide feedback for healthy and successful living. Likewise, at the work place, it is natural to expect guidance and feedback from supervisors and fellow workers. Even negative feedback provides recognition of one's existence within the organization.

Regular feedback, like the sun, provides light in order to guide the worker toward the type of performance that is satisfying to the self as well as to recipients of the service. Also, like the rays of the sun, feedback must be regular and nourishing or individuals will not grow and become optimally productive. In addition to the worker's need to receive feedback is the supervisor's need for the time and ability to provide it. If a superior is overwhelmed with work and large numbers of people to supervise, he or she will never have the opportunity to provide guidance. Resentment and apathy mount and production lags as worker recognition decreases. Although an appropriate "pat on the back" is more nourishing than a reprimand, both stimulate awareness and a chance to reflect upon one's performance.

Like other workers, an educator wants to know the expectations of the organization, the behaviors that will be successful or unsuccessful in satisfying job requirements, any physical and psychological dangers that might exist, and the security of the job. Education employees need feedback to develop job values, aspirations, objectives, and accomplishments. Lack of clear, consistent information can result in distress. There are many uncertainties (fiscal problems, technological breakthroughs that eliminate jobs, declining enrollment, possible reduction of staff) that lead to perceived anticipatory stress.

The greatest need for feedback concerns the immediate consequence of one's actions. If evaluations only happen once or twice a year without regular, periodic feedback, the possibility of stress increases the longer the employee works in a vacuum. The withholding of information from the worker creates dislike and distrust, as well as a lack of confidence in superiors and the organization as a whole. Some of the more significant research findings are reported here:

- Kasl (1973) found that low job satisfaction was related to the inability of supervisors to provide feedback and the lack of recognition for good performance.
- Erez (1977) indicated that certain job information was absolutely necessary for personal comfort, recognition, and direction.
- Kim (1975) found that feedback and goals are interactively related to performance. His study supports others' findings that knowledge alone is not sufficient for effective performance. He found that attainment of goals was significantly higher when feedback was provided. Kim clearly showed that work behavior can be changed directly without going through the process of attitude change. Feedback given to workers focused on observable tasks and affected positive job performance. Although job satisfaction was less affected by feedback, job performance was improved significantly.
- Pritchard and Montagno (1978) found significantly increased productivity when feedback on performance was provided.
- Koch (1976) found not only a significantly higher level of productivity, but product quality was increased while turnover and absenteeism decreased when feedback was provided by supervisors.

Education and other helping professions have a unique problem with feedback. Frequently the recipients of services express their dissatisfaction and rarely provide positive feedback. Instead, a taken-for-granted approach ("that's what you're getting paid for") takes away the satisfaction of knowing you have been helpful. If recipients do not provide some positive feedback, negative attitudes toward one's job can develop. Under these conditions motivation decreases, productivity slows, and distance (psychological insulation) increases between professional and recipient. When effectiveness is impaired, it becomes easy for the professional to blame recipients for being "unmotivated," unwilling, and inherently at fault for their lack of progress or continued problems.

Conversely, Dr. Hans Selye stated (Proctor, 1979), "Successful people live longer. There's an anti-stress effect in success. Very great painters, very great scientists and very great actors are extremely long lived." Other concomitant factors such as security, social recognition, and the opportunity to take time off when the job gets overwhelming also contribute to a reduction of stress among the famous. The positive feedback that successful people receive is highly nourishing.

Communication.   The work place is frequently a social system in itself, characterized by the nature of its interpersonal relationships. A work environment can provide an opportunity for social support and friendship beyond the sphere of work. Job satisfaction is enhanced by friendly relationships, and task interdependence complements social interaction.

Individuals who express high job satisfaction indicate that they are able to communicate openly with supervisors, fellow employees, and recipients of their services or products. When intense feelings arise, these people are able to express themselves rather than repress their emotions. Feelings kept inside create physical and emotional stress, which in turn has a direct effect upon productivity and job satisfaction. Organizational structures that support open, honest, cathartic expression in a positive and constructive way reap large dividends from employees. Interestingly enough, it has been found that when management reacts to open communication on a crisis basis only, it reinforces negative communications.

Good working relationships and communication with fellow workers are significant factors in occupational and individual health. Some significant studies are reported as follows:

- Argyris (1971), Cooper and Marshall (1976), Herzberg (1966), and many others have found that poor interpersonal relationships can cause significant distress among workers. Lack of trust, lack of cooperation, or lack of support are all considered significant causes of occupational distress.
- Imberman's study (1976) emphasized the importance of communication in organizations. He said that the four major complaints in industry are (1) the work environment, (2) misunderstanding of policy, (3) harsh, abusive, or inept supervision, and (4) sins of omission (failure to provide feedback).
- Downs (1973), through a factor analytic study, found "communication climate" and "communication with superiors" as ultimately important to job holders.

In order to counter these complaints, Imberman strongly suggests that communication (listening and addressing issues) (1) provides constructive criticism instead of wasted resources and indirect criticism; (2) provides favorable and genuine management concern by lowering absenteeism and turnover, reducing waste, and improving quality and productivity; and (3) prevents future problems. An environment of clear, open communication avoids negative retribution.

Opportunity for employees to communicate increases peer support. Frequent communication with fellow employees provides a means to share similar personal concerns. Lack of regular contact can induce social withdrawal. Regular communication tends to prevent or forestall the onset of burnout.

Research data strongly support the fact that people need someone they can trust and with whom they can communicate. Having a confidant or "supportive other" assists in short-circuiting the effects of distress. Similar research with families and couples supports the positive effects of good communication and its direct relationship with successful living. It is fair to say that life is not complete unless it allows for intimacy with others. This is only accomplished through good communication.

Work Overload or Underload

Researchers have found high levels of stress among individuals who have had excessive work loads. Long or unpredictable hours, too many responsibilities, work at a too-rapid pace, too many phone calls, dealing directly with difficult people without sufficient relief, dealing with constant crises, and supervising too many people or having broad, multifaceted job descriptions are characteristics of work overload. In recent years some data have surfaced regarding boring, tedious jobs or jobs without variety as being equally distressful. As in most elements of nature, compromise between boredom and overload appears to be the most healthy.

Work overload or underload can be divided into three categories:

Psychological—frustration caused by the employee's inability to cope with job ambiguity or interactions with people at work.

Physical—distress caused by too much or too little physical exercise on the job; work conditions such as crowded offices, monotonous jobs, or fluctuation from crisis to boredom (firemen, police, lab technicians).

Social—social pressure placed upon employees (peer pressure, uncommunicative fellow workers, or social expectations).

Obviously, if an employee is bombarded by the frustration and demands of the supervisor and recipients of services rendered (psychological), works in a small, dark, cold office (physical), or is ostracized by fellow employees (social), the chances of burnout increase significantly.

- Kahn (1973) found that the most common complaint among professionals is work overload.
- Sales (1970) found that those who reported greater work overload were found to have higher levels of job-related tension.
- French and Caplan (1973) determined that greater overload brought about lower levels of self-esteem, higher blood cholesterol, and faster heart rates.
- Rogers (1975, 1977) found work load the most frequent cause of stress in managers. (Other major distressors included organizational structure or design, responsibility, communication, and interpersonal interaction.)

Using a somewhat different breakdown, French and Caplan (1973) have differentiated work overload in terms of quantitative and qualitative characteristics. Quantitative overload refers to having "just too much to do" while qualitative overload refers to "very difficult work." Their research indicates that in combination, quantitative and qualitative work overload produce nine different stress symptoms: psychological and physical strain, job dissatisfaction, job tension, lower self-esteem, psychological threat, embarrassment, high cholesterol levels, increased heart rate, and more smoking.

Quantitative overload.   Quantitative overload includes the volume of tasks necessary to successfully complete an assignment.

- Caplan et al. (1975) found the amount of unwanted overtime and the employee's perception of quantitative work overload to be significantly related to psychological stress. The effects of quantitative work overload are primarily evidenced by signs of depression, anxiety, and irritation.
- Breslow and Buell (1960) reported that a relationship existed between hours worked and coronary disease. They found that California light-industry employees under the age of 45 who worked more than 48 hours a week had twice the risk of death from heart attacks than their counterparts working 40 hours or less per week.
- Terryberry (1968) found that quantitative overload in most organizations led to a breakdown of physical health.
- Margolis et al. (1974) using a national sample found quantitative overload related to drinking problems, absenteeism, low motivation, and lowered self-esteem. (Although statistically significant, the relationships were very small.)

- Cooper and Marshall (1976), Quinn, Seashore, and Mangione (1971), and Porter and Lawler (1965) felt that quantitative overload, although a potential source of occupational stress, was not by itself a main factor in occupational disease. Cooper and Marshall expressed their strong suspicion that qualitative overload (difficult work) was more significant than the amount of work.

Qualitative overload.   The most qualitatively difficult task and occupational stressor is "responsibility for people."

- Wardwell, Hyman, and Bahnson (1970) in a comparison of individuals—those who have responsibility for things (equipment, supplies), and those who are responsible for people—found that responsibility for people was significantly more likely to lead to heart disease and other indices of distress such as high blood pressure.
- French and Caplan (1970) and Wardwell et al. found that responsibility for people rather than things led to a higher rate of heart attack and was related to heavy smoking, diastolic blood pressure, and high cholesterol levels.

Responsibility for people is an awesome assignment. It involves interacting with others, evaluating, giving reprimands and praise, directing meetings, keeping others informed, completing reports, composing memos, mediating interpersonal conflicts, accountability for the behavior of others, crisis intervention, and the continual need for providing support, understanding, and assistance. Each individual has a different personality, abilities, and experiences, and therefore deserves personal attention. The person who assumes responsibility for the safety and lives of others assumes a tremendous work load.

- Wahlund and Nerell (1977) found that administrators, teachers, engineers, and police fall within a high mental-stress group. Seven times as many members of these professions reported lacking time to complete their duties, as compared to a low mental-stress group. Wahlund and Nerell found that the major factors causing mental strain at work, in rank order, were heavy responsibility (especially for people), shortage of time, excessive work load, and the demands and expectations of outsiders.
- Pincherle (1972) found evidence of physical stress linked to age and level of responsibility of managers—the older and more responsible the manager, the greater the presence of cardiovascular disease.
- Terhune (1963) and Eaton (1969) found similar relationships among age, responsibility, and stress-related illness. They reported that as

one gets older, lack of resistance to stress and its cumulative effects might increase stress-related disease.

- French and Caplan (1970) found that responsibility for people was significantly related to heavy smoking, diastolic blood pressure, and serum cholesterol levels. The more the individual had responsibility for things as opposed to people, the lower were each of these cardiovascular disease factors.
- Friedman, Rosenman, and Carroll (1958) and Dreyfuss and Czackes (1959) have also reported the potential of heart disease characterized by increased cholesterol levels in victims of qualitative work overload.

Research has clearly shown that the qualitative overload of unpredictable changes or crises causes more distress than predictable change. School administrators, air traffic controllers, police, and others who face a constant barrage of unpredictable change have noticeably higher distress-related symptoms. School officials have frequently reported increased anxiety and discomfort in the face of upcoming initiative elections or pending legislation that portends unknown changes in their jobs. Their fear is that within a relatively short period of time, large amounts of new and unpredictable change will be required of them.

Since the difficulty of each individual's work is to a degree relative and subjective, reliable studies in this area are lacking. Anecdoctal data from workers suffering from burnout, however, strongly support qualitative work overload as a significant occupational stressor.

Contact Overload

Contact overload results from the necessity for frequent encounters with other people in order to carry out job functions. Some occupations (teaching, counseling, law enforcement) require many encounters that are unpleasant and therefore distressful. These workers—frequently professional—spend a large proportion of their work time interacting with people in various states of distress. Client state-of-mind contributes significantly to the reactions of the helper; it is as if some of the client's bad feelings can rub off on the professional. Physicians have the highest rate (10 percent) of alcoholism of any profession; psychiatrists have a higher suicide rate than any other profession; school administrators have an alarming rate of ulcers and heart attacks. Bank tellers and others who transact routinely with huge numbers of customers are exposed to contact overload; yet they have minimal stress reactions, because of limited emotional demands made upon them.

It has been demonstrated that professional helpers need to have adequate time to provide necessary care. If the caseload is too large, too little time is available for quality services. If personal attention is lacking, clients are more easily referred to abstractly as "cases" or "files." With an increased caseload comes a constant stream of direct contacts that leaves little time for rest and reflection. When the caseload is high, control over one's work and consequent job satisfaction is affected. Contact overload also leaves little occasion or energy for communication and support from fellow employees or for seeking personal and professional growth opportunities.

- Colligan, Smith, and Hurrell (1977) found that health care professionals exhibited the highest incidence of mental disorder admissions. In explaining these results, they found that the responsibility of caring for and interacting with people who are ill or infirm can be emotionally demanding, thus subjecting the health professional to considerable distress.
- Freudenberger (1975) and Mattingly (1977) have found that direct contact with children and parents creates cognitive overload. Added to the intensity of interaction, this massive overload affects employee performance; decision-making problems and greater emotional insulation result.
- Maslach and Pines (1977) found that as the number of clients a professional serves increases, the general result is greater cognitive, sensory, and emotional overload. However, the data reveal that longer working hours (a quantitative factor) are correlated with higher stress and negative staff attitudes only when they involve continuous direct contact with clients.

Perhaps the most common phenomenon in working with difficult and needy people is the "rescuer syndrome." Usually it is based on the helper's assumption that the recipient is incapable of doing something for him- or herself, or that it is easier to assume the responsibility for the needy person. Helping others may be the American way, but it breeds dependency, takes away the rights and responsibilities of others, and robs them of self-esteem. Rescuing also drains the professional and results in psychological exhaustion. If a disproportionately high level of psychological energy is expended by the professional while a low amount is required of the recipient, exhaustion of the helper results. It is most important to realize that although people may appreciate a guiding hand, they'd rather do it themselves. Help needs to be in a form of educational guidance. Galileo said it well: "You can't teach man anything, you can only help him to discover it for himself."

The emotional pressure of working closely with difficult and needy people is a continual stressor. Helping professionals wear away gradually under the never-ending onslaught of distress. As the number of supervisors, fellow workers, and recipients of one's work increases, the amount of distress increases geometrically rather than linearly. Research in the area of helping professions shows that as caseloads become high, burnout increases. In industry, as production demands increase beyond a reasonable level, job turnover and physical complaints become disproportionately high. However, research data strongly support the fact that professionals having direct contact with difficult people experience significantly greater distress than those having contact with things.

Role Conflict/Ambiguity

No individual can be all things to all people, especially today. Because of societal demands, increased technology, changes in the family, and a lack of trust in institutions, the typical job in today's industrial society has become more complicated, technical, political, and tenuous than ever before. Job descriptions are replete with major responsibilities that demand extensive pretraining, as well as ongoing inservice. The areas of expected specialization are vast, and the pressure to be an expert in several areas is sometimes overwhelming.

Although role conflict and role ambiguity may occur independently of one another, they both refer to the uncertainty about what one is expected to do at work. Role conflict deals with the expectations of people involved with work, while role ambiguity deals with the nature and degree of those expectations. Both produce distress and lower job satisfaction, and both result in less trust and confidence in others. They both limit the worker's authority and create strained communication.

Role conflict. Role conflict may be defined as the simultaneous occurrence of two or more opposing pressures such that a response to one makes compliance with the other impossible. It is exemplified by being torn between groups expecting different kinds of behavior. For example, a superintendent may hold a school principal responsible to carry out organizational policies "by the book." At the same time, the teacher may exert pressure for a more flexible, relaxed approach that provides for more autonomy and localized decision making. The pressures from above and below are obviously incompatible and in distinct conflict. Research literature is replete with case histories of middle managers as victims of this double-bind conflict. The most frequent role conflicts are (1) those between the individual's values and those of a superior or the organization; (2) the conflict between the demands of the work place and the worker's personal life; and (3) the conflict between worker abilities and organizational expectations.

- McGrath (1970a) and Kraut (1965) found that the results of role conflict include low job satisfaction, frustration, decreased trust and respect, low confidence in the organization, morale problems, and high degrees of tension. The most frequent response to role conflict is withdrawal and nonresolution of problems. According to McGrath, the highest incidence of role conflict exists at the middle levels of management (school principals, departmental chairpersons, program directors). He strongly suggested close, positive, interpersonal relationships among all members and levels of an organization as the only means of resolving role conflicts.
- Kahn et al. (1964) found that high role-conflict employees suffered lower job satisfaction and higher job-related tension. Role conflict was discovered to be a major source of psychological stress. The researchers determined that the greater the authority of the people issuing the conflicting role messages, the more job dissatisfaction was produced by role conflict.
- Caplan and Jones (1975) reported low job satisfaction when job ambiguity was high. They also found increased blood pressure and heart rate.
- Margolis et al. (1974) discovered a significant relationship between high job ambiguity and negative mood, lowered self-esteem, job dissatisfaction, low motivation, and intention to leave the job.
- Shirom et al. (1973) found a highly significant relationship between role conflict and abnormal electrocardiograph readings for white-collar workers. Their study found that as workers move from blue-collar to white-collar jobs (clerical, managerial, or professional), there is an increased likelihood of occupational stress caused by role conflict.
- Caplan et al. (1975) found role conflict to be the stress variable most highly correlated with irritation, a measure of psychological stress. In addition, role conflict correlated more consistently with anxiety and depression than did any other stress variable. It was the only stressor to correlate significantly with somatic complaints. Another interesting finding was that mistrust of fellow workers related positively to high role ambiguity, and the condition led to inadequate communication, psychological stress, and low job satisfaction.

- Cherniss, Egnatios, and Wacker (1976) found that role conflict was especially strong for new public professionals. They pointed to two factors in particular that seem to have close relationship to this conflict: the social change and ferment that have occurred in all professions during the last 15 years, and the challenge of existing in a bureaucracy while trying to provide a human service.
- Mattingly (1977), in her discussion of the sources of burnout in child care workers, pointed to the inevitable role conflict involved in child care practice. She stated that even in agencies that maintain moderate or better standards of care, there is an ongoing conflict between client care and custodial and managerial requirements. Mattingly believes that this conflict seems likely to be experienced more acutely as professional child care workers have decreasing participation in the decision-making bodies of agencies.
- Freudenberger (1975), in discussing burnout among administrators, cited a very real cause to be the fact that the administrator is constantly having to "change hats." The many roles in which he or she must function, some of them conflicting, can be a potential source of distress.

Role ambiguity.   Role ambiguity may be defined as a lack of clarity about the job, that is, a discrepancy between the information available to the employee and that which is required for successful job performance. The phenomenon is frequently seen in occupations with high technological or political change.

In addition to the research studies reported above, an additional reference should be cited.

- Abdel-Halim (1978) found that in comparison to role conflict and work overload, role ambiguity had the highest correlation to job dissatisfaction. He also found, however, that it is very difficult to provide enough role clarity for administrators without introducing unnecessary structure or rigidity to the work itself.

School administrators are frequently unclear about the scope of their job. They simply do not know where it begins and where it ends. This occurs especially when job requirements become ever-expanding, and they must face continually greater demands from the public.

NON-ORGANIZATIONAL CAUSES

Individual Factors

Obviously everyone entering the world of work does not arrive with the same intellectual, physical, psychological, and socioeconomic background. Researchers have found that family problems (Pahl & Pahl, 1971; Dohrenwend & Dohrenwend, 1974) and other individual factors do affect tolerance and reaction to stress. The interaction between private life (family, finances) and work life is a topic upon which research data is lacking. The mutual interaction and accumulation of both personal and occupational stressors can certainly contribute to job burnout. A worker burdened by the death of a parent, an impending divorce, or concern about difficulties at work is a strong candidate for job burnout.

Personality factors. Stress at the work place is not equally damaging to all who experience it. Extensive research has been conducted on personality variables. Kahn et al. (1964) have identified a number of personality types who appear to be more susceptible to occupational stress.

Neuroticism: One is the neurotic, a person characterized by emotional instability and low self-confidence. Neurotics contribute to an organization by throwing themselves into their jobs with a vengeance; yet, because they are anxiety prone, they tend to worry needlessly and succumb to stress. The remarkable memory for detail, analytic ability, and overpreparedness of neurotics are beneficial to the organization, but exact a cost on themselves and their families. Interestingly, the presence of environmental stress seems to produce neurotic emotional reactions in those who originally scored low on the neurotic anxiety scale (Kahn et al., 1964).

Introversion: Another personality dimension that has received a great deal of attention is extroversion-introversion. It has been documented that the outgoing person has a better capacity to deal with stress.

The introverted personality, although capable of close personal relationships, tends under stress conditions to reduce social contacts. The introvert's problem-solving or coping techniques are based upon withdrawal from stress. This, in turn, causes isolation, antisocial behavior, and begins a cycle that results in even greater sensitivity to stress.

Flexibility: Flexible individuals are characterized as open-minded, democratic, and other-directed. This personality is in contrast to the rigid individual who is close-minded, dogmatic, authoritarian, and inner-directed. The rigid individual prefers well-defined, stable, and hierarchical levels of organization, while the flexible individual prefers equality, change, cultivation of new ideas, and variability of experience. Unfortunately, flexible people expose themselves to more stress by not being able to say no. They frequently promise more than they are able to deliver. Some researchers have likened flexible vs. rigid personality traits to the democratic vs. autocratic continuum. Democratic/flexible persons are more prone to organizational stress than their autocratic/rigid counterparts.

Status Orientation: The status-oriented person is an individual who is striving, highly involved in work, independent, and seeking advancement. The security-oriented individual by contrast is more dependent, worries about job stability, wants to be liked by others, and attributes power to others. The organizational environment is more hostile to the status oriented than the security oriented. Status-oriented people react strongly to job conflicts and more easily succumb to stress.

Sex differences.   Researchers have begun to study the response differences that exist between sexes.

- In a study funded by the National Institute for Mental Health, Lieberman and Pearlin (1979) identified ten major sources of general distress among Chicagoans in their roles as workers, spouses, and parents. Half of the sources of distress were related to occupation. Significantly more applied to women than to men. Women were found to be more likely to be laid off, fired, or to voluntarily give up employment. Women were also more likely than men to find jobs unrewarding, while men were more often found to be exposed to pressures and depersonalizing experiences on the job.
- The results of a study by Simpe (1975) indicated that job-related strain could be effectively predicted using a combination of job and life stresses. For males, "under-utilization of abilities" and "lack of participation" job stressors accounted for more of the effect of total strain than life stress. For females, life stress accounted for more of the variance in strain than any of the job stresses. It was also found that females had significantly higher life-stress levels than males.
- Puff and Moeckel (1979) found that women in management positions faced the same stressors as men, but they were also victims of additional stressors. Women were more negatively affected by conflicts between their social, family, and work roles.
- Hollon and Gemmill (1976) found that female teaching professionals reported experiencing less participation in decision making, less job involvement, less job satisfaction, and more job-related tension than their male counterparts.
- Chronic excessive stress/distress causes a sharp decrease in the level

of a male's primary hormone, testosterone, which has a direct influence upon sex drive. Men constantly in a state of moderate to severe stress lose their drive to perform sex. A study of Vietnam soldiers (Lamott, 1975) under stress found urine samples contained abnormally low levels of testosterone. When not in stress situations it was found that these same men's testosterone levels rose dramatically. It has been shown that sperm counts also decrease under significant stress conditions. Women have also been found to suffer a reduction in sex hormones (progesterone) when under prolonged stress. With decreased levels of progesterone, women frequently experience menstrual irregularities that can cause other physical problems. Researchers have also found dysfunctional sex problems when either men or women were exposed to prolonged stress.

Other individual factors and studies.   Researchers have carried out a number of studies that give possible explanations for increased stress and heart disease.

- Schafer (1978) found that certain general categories of people are more likely to encounter distress. These include: (1) divorced, unhappily married, or unmarried; (2) recent widows and widowers; (3) families who move a great deal; (4) the unemployed and poor; (5) black men; and (6) urban dwellers.
- Levine (1967 & 1975) has shown in laboratory studies that animals subjected to stress (electrical shock) early in their lives developed normally and were able to cope well with later stress. However, those that received no such aversive stimulation grew up to be timid and less adaptive in adult life. It may thus be that a person's response to stress is similarly related to the nature of his or her early environment. Perhaps individual differences in response to stress are more related to early exposure and possible preventive conditioning than to innate or hereditary factors.
- Jenkins (1971), in an extensive review of studies, revealed that fatal heart disease increases when individuals show greater emotional instability (especially depression), have high anxiety scores, and tend to be introverted. Jenkins also found that those who were so deeply committed to their work they neglected other aspects of their lives had significantly higher incidence of heart disease.
- Drs. Friedman and Rosenman (1974) found that individuals who were highly competitive, aggressive, impatient, tense, and restless (Type A) were significantly more subject to heart attacks. It thus appears that the personality one brings to the work place contributes to cardiovascular disease.

It would appear that persons who are more neurotic, introverted, flexible/democratic, status and achievement oriented are significantly more susceptible to stress than those who are more emotionally stable, extroverted, rigid/autocratic, and security oriented. Realistically, few people fall at the extremes of these continuums; instead, most individuals fall somewhere within the middle of each range of personality characteristics. The implication of the research is that people react to various levels of stress on the basis of their complex, individual personality type.

At this point it may be helpful to differentiate job burnout from cardiovascular disease or mental dysfunction. The excessive stressors of burnout affect all personality types, particularly those who manifest less adaptive coping skills and thus are more vulnerable to burnout. However, distress at extreme levels is indiscriminate. It does not seem to matter if one is aggressive or submissive, extroverted or introverted, Type A or B, active or passive, healthy or neurotic. On the contrary, it seems to more seriously affect those who when hired are genuinely conscientious, intelligent, hard working, interested, competent, and physically healthy.

Job frustration can perhaps be best described as the generic cause of burnout. Frustration is caused by lack of communication, poor feedback, limited participation in decision making, and other factors. Burnout appears to be principally caused by one's job stressors. Cardiovascular problems, on the other hand, appear to be primarily related to an individual predisposition (especially personality) and only secondarily related to other stressors (job factors) that aggravate the condition.

Training Deficits

Several different areas of job training are necessary to prevent occupational distress. The most obvious area is adequate initial preparation. Training and competencies are necessary to bolster confidence, as well as to allow the worker to get through each day without unnecessary dependence upon others or upon reference materials. On-the-job training is also necessary as technology advances. New professionals are most susceptible to some forms of distress.

- According to Cherniss, Egnatios, and Wacker (1976), there seem to be two major training deficits that affect new public professionals. First, with the possible exception of mental health workers, public professionals do not study the helping process and their own role in it. A professional's role involves working with individuals or groups in a helping relationship. Yet, very little training is devoted to learning this helping process. A second aspect of role performance that is often neglected is how to negotiate one's way through bureaucracy. For example, public school teachers must learn to acquire needed supplies through a system that is frequently complicated. Public defenders must learn the intricacies of plea bargaining, and other courtroom skills. New professionals are often ill prepared in understanding the helping process and maneuvering within the public organization. Until skill is mastered in these areas, distress can be severe.

• Almost every research study dealing with occupational distress cites the need for a balance among resources, including the training of individuals for the demands of the job (Albrecht, 1979; Argyris, 1971; Caplan et al., 1975; Cooper & Marshall, 1975; Freudenberger, 1975; Kahn & Quinn, 1970; Lazarus, 1966; Maslach, 1977; Mattingly, 1977; Wahlund & Nerell, 1977).

Secondly, training in communication skills is necessary in order to facilitate the ability of the employee to relate successfully with supervisors, fellow workers, and recipients of services or products. According to one survey, jobs are more frequently lost because of poor communication than because of any other factor.

Finally, one needs to be taught how to deal with stress. Everyone needs to learn methods of coping with the variety of stressors faced each day. Unfortunately, few institutions or job-training programs provide any semblance of preparation for stress. We are inoculated against relatively rare diseases, but seldom is attention paid to a much more mortal enemy—distress. Coping, a survival skill against distress, appears to be at least as important as any other job-related training. Coping involves understanding the ubiquitousness of stress, personal control, tolerance for ambiguity, personal awareness, relaxation techniques, individual strategies, and practice under simulated conditions.

SECONDARY CAUSES OF JOB BURNOUT

Job burnout is caused by multiple stressors of both primary and secondary natures. Secondary stressors are those occupational or personal elements that further add to the effect of previously existing stressors and tip the balance toward distress. A review of common secondary factors indicates that relationship.

Societal Changes

According to Albrecht (1979) changes in society since 1900 have been startling, bewildering, and sometimes alarming. In 1900 only 39 percent of the population lived in urban areas, while today almost 75 percent occupies our major metropolitan areas. This migration has changed the life style of a huge number of Americans; most people are now directly or indirectly dependent upon others. Living in close proximity to those whom we know only casually creates an oppressive physical and psychological milieu. Fighting traffic and crowds, living in a compressed environment, and acting as a social unit typifies our new society. Crime and violence terrify old and young alike. The frenetic pace of life keeps our minds and bodies in a constant state of arousal virtually unknown in 1900.

With the revolution in transportation, man has become dramatically more mobile. Job relocation has become a common phenomenon. What was once a typical sequence of being born, living, and dying in a single community has essentially disappeared. A more common pattern today involves multiple relocations for educational, occupational, and other reasons. If someone were to propose to the typical citizen of 1890 that a new discovery would soon be available that would assist in travel, farming, and pleasure alike, yet guarantee 50,000 deaths each year, it would be difficult to believe that the citizen would support such "newfangled nonsense" as the automobile in the name of progress.

Changes in family life in the past few decades have had a significant effect upon the social functions of work. The scattering of large families in various localities has resulted in less emotional support and more isolation. Physical separation reduces the opportunity to call upon the extended family for support and understanding—both of which are defenses against stress. Consequently, many people turn to the work place to find a potentially major social support system. Many industries have extensive social and recreational activities to assuage the effects of distance and remoteness of kin.

Information Overload

So much information has been made available through the mass media that the public is now being deluged with information overload. We are notified within minutes about morbid crimes, disasters, and crises. The reports are multitudinous and in distressing detail. The accounts are intended to catch public attention, and in fact, they do so to such an extent that some individuals react with emotional fervor. Anxieties are increased and burdens are added to our already overloaded stress defense systems.

The power of media persuasion, particularly that of television, is formidable. Some 96 percent of households in the United States have a television set, and each person averages about four hours per day watching highly influential material. It has been predicted that today's youth and tomorrow's adults will obtain their primary values from television. Many children already have a distorted view of the incidence of violence and crime in our society. It is the opinion of many that the media overload the public with information about problems beyond the viewers' direct control. The exposure to societal ills outside the viewers' ability to control can create unnecessary fears.

This knowledge explosion has been expanded by advanced technology. Few of us are able to read every journal, magazine, or book we receive. The more we learn the more we realize how much more there is to learn. Each significant new piece of information creates the need for more information. Even the use of advanced computer technology does not provide a final answer to data management; indeed the computer sometimes compounds the problem by generating additional information or the need to view data from different perspectives. Input overload can be a real problem in many jobs. The problem of dissemination—let alone the need for analysis and verification—can create overload stress.

Life-style Changes

Our life-style has been a sedentary one. The United States now needs only 4 percent of its population to grow farm products. Most jobs that develop as the need for agricultural workers decreases require more mental than physical exertion. Many individuals now lack physical exercise and are more prone to psychological stress and physical ailments. Physically active individuals tend to handle stress more efficiently than their sedentary counterparts.

Our American society, although one of the most comfortable in the world, has had to pay a price for its success. By living at a fast pace, in crowded conditions, being highly mobile, generally sedentary, and bombarded by information overload, we have created a new set of stresses with which our bodies are unfamiliar and against which our somatic and psychological defense systems are unprepared.

Medical research and treatment have all but eliminated most of yesteryear's fatal or disabling diseases, yet there has been an increase in the incidence of distress-related diseases (Benson, 1975; Stoyva,

1976). Within the past three-quarters of a century, we have seen heart attacks increase by over 340 percent. Over one million Americans have heart attacks each year, and hypertension kills some 60,000 people yearly. Another problem linked to distress is alcoholism. James Schreier (Albrecht, 1979, pp. 32–34) of Marquette University concluded that alcoholism alone costs the American society about $15 billion a year. He also believes that the abuse of various other drugs may cost society another $15 billion.

Lack of Confidence in Institutions

Business, government, labor, religious institutions, professions, and the military recently have all fallen in the general public esteem. Respect for authority has proportionally declined. Mistrust in the presidency, as well as in most American institutions, has reached epidemic proportions. For example, lack of trust in big business had risen from 30 percent in 1968 to 70 percent in 1975. In fact by 1975, 90 percent of American citizens expressed general mistrust of those in power. Until the mid 1960s, most institutions enjoyed a relatively positive image. The decline of public support and confidence in education, together with the decline of the family, church, and community, have put additional pressure upon the public schools.

Job Security

The feeling of job security depends upon the predictability, feedback, and friendliness inherent in the work environment. Obviously, the employee will feel more secure in the job if information is provided regularly and is reliable. Another aspect of job security is the degree of acceptance and understanding a person experiences from colleagues. When one works with individuals who provide reassurance, trust, and support, full attention and energy can be focused upon work objectives. Conversely, when one is preoccupied with job insecurity, he or she is apt to worry and dissipate energy needed for optimal work effectiveness.

Setting Limits

Most jobs provide employees with an opportunity to work as long and hard as they desire. Educators have been used to accepting more and more assignments without regard to possible overload. As physical and psychological limits are approached, saying no becomes necessary to avoid overextending our finite ability to respond. Setting reasonable limits conserves both time and energy. Each individual must determine his or her energy output limit. Avoiding unnecessary energy consumption in the form of physical and mental distress is reminiscent of a popular oil filter advertisement narrated by a mechanic who says, "You can pay me now [for an oil filter] or pay me later [for a completely rebuilt engine]."

Mid-Career Phenomena

Mid-career stress is associated exclusively with the middle-aged individual and his or her job. The response to anxieties is often directed toward the work place and occurs more frequently at the midpoint of life, when the reality of success (or lack of success) is most critical. There are relatively few research studies of the mid-career stage that objectively and systematically define this potential crisis period. Only recently has there been acknowledgment of the unique phenomena that occur in middle age. It used to be assumed that once within the work force, a person would not change. Today there are many workers in mid-career status—the range of age from 35-55 years. Individuals in this age range are subject to many pressures. The work place occupies a focal point for the middle aged in terms of their expectations and success, but the mid-career worker is subject as well to social and family pressures.

One research study (Thompson & Dalton, 1976) found a negative correlation between age and performance after age 35. Their study indicated that mid-life crisis (age obsolescence) need not be inevitable nor the major determinant of poor performance. They found that some professionals remain high performers throughout their long careers. The critical areas that appeared to determine performance were not age but on-the-job activities. Thompson and Dalton stated the belief that organizational obsolescence, not age obsolescence, is the main culprit to performance drops after age 35. More effective organizations have policies and practices that help professionals move through various stages of development and responsibility. This contrasts with less effective organizations that hinder professional development and movement, and actually contribute to age obsolescence. Over the past two decades many organizations have attempted to combat this problem by creating dual avenues of recognition—one a specialized technical avenue and the other a management route—both of which offer opportunities for increased salary and status. Organizations are beginning to pay for outstanding individual performance regardless of position, thereby financially rewarding technical contributions and not just management responsibility. Extensive further study will be necessary to determine the effect of this phenomenon upon the worker.

Physical and Mental Exhaustion

When a person begins to experience distress, be it organizational or personal, the body and mind send out ominous signals. There is a tendency to become fatigued, there is difficulty in concentrating and sleeping, headaches or stomach problems develop, or the person is simply not operating at full capability. Employees are not generally encouraged to leave work unless they show physical symptoms of illness. Consequently, bodies and minds may reach a point of exhaustion before there is any palliative action. Our medical and insurance companies pay our bills only if we are sick. Dr. C. Norman Shealley has found that 50 percent of all hospital patients are there because the insurance company only pays for hospital admissions. Negative reinforcements abound when it comes to health: health insurers and organizations reimburse only when people are sick; no payments or dividends are provided when people are able to maintain their health. Perhaps a revised process might be developed where "well days" are allocated to reward the worker for not getting sick, rather than the current emphasis on sickness and medical dependence.

Most employees find vacation a welcome relief and a time for healthy distractions. Likewise a "mental health day" or "time out" could periodically provide a chance to recharge one's batteries. No one has all perfect days, weeks, years. It is not only in the interest of the worker that an occasional "well day" be taken when needed—the practice is of benefit to the recipients of services as well. Teachers, firemen, or air traffic controllers, for instance, may bring physical or mental injury to others if they force themselves to work when they are not fit and alert. One mistake can be very costly.

Underutilization of Skills

Many new professionals enter work life freshly trained and full of idealistic expectations. Some of them are jarred by the realization of their limited effect upon the organization, but there is another phenomenon common among highly trained beginning workers which can be equally disturbing. The under-utilization of an individual's skills can be so stultifying as to create distress. If, for example, a teacher is both trained and naturally skilled in one subject area, but is required to teach a different subject instead, frustration can result. The frustration of not being able to utilize chosen areas of study can diminish enthusiasm and productivity. In periods of declining school enrollment, educational specialists (art or music teachers, counselors, nurses, librarians) may find themselves assigned to duties almost totally alien from their areas of specialized training. Likewise, a lack of recognition of workers' special abilities or interests can cause them to suffer job dissatisfaction and poor morale. Self-esteem is an important psychological factor that is essential to the success of all professionals.

Physical Work Conditions

Working in an environment that provides little space, inadequate light, insufficient temperature control, excessive noise, poor equipment, or limited supplies will have a direct effect upon job satisfaction and productivity. Space that is personal, has adequate ventilation and light, is well-equipped and quiet, provides health-enhancing conditions for employees. Employee satisfaction is not only a reflection of their respect for supervisory personnel and the organization, but also of their comfort in the place where they work.

SUMMARY

More research will be necessary to determine the specific impact of various stressors, particularly the interplay between organizational and non-organizational causes. An extensive review of the literature makes it clear that a number of identified factors do indeed contribute to occupational distress and job burnout. Work environments in modern organizations have significant impact upon physical and mental health. The identification of stressors aids us in taking the steps necessary to alleviate both physical and mental risks of occupationally related disease.

Job satisfaction is engendered when working conditions include adequate training, reasonable responsibility, limitations on direct contact with needy people, supportive supervision, enhancing feedback, good communication, positive attitudes on the part of both management and employees, opportunities for new ideas, and limited job ambiguity. We know that as productivity increases, absenteeism and turnover decrease, and morale is optimal. Obviously, the hiring of individuals with limited life skills or family problems contributes to organizational distress. However, it is the responsibility of the organization—as well as the individual—to try to alleviate negative factors affecting employee well-being and productivity and to make positive the quality of inter-action between the individual and the organization.

Christina Maslach (1977) has written,*

> Although personality variables of individuals are not irrelevant in our overall analysis of burnout, I am forced by the weight of my research data to conclude that the problem is best understood in terms of the social and situational sources of job related stress. The prevalence of the phenomenon and the range of seemingly disparate professionals who are affected by it suggest that the search for causes is better directed away from the unending cycle of identifying "bad people" and toward uncovering the operational and structural characteristics in the "bad" situations where many good people function. We have reached the point at which the number of rotten apples in the barrel warrants an examination of the barrel itself. (p. 14)

---

* Used by permission of Christina Maslach, from "Burn-out: A Social Psychological Analysis" (paper presented at the A.P.A. Convention, August 1977). To be published in J. W. Jones (Ed.), *The Burnout Syndrome* (Chicago: London House Press, in press).

CHAPTER IV

Bureaucracy,
Job Satisfaction, and Job Turnover

BUREAUCRACY

Bureaucracy is defined in *Webster's New World Dictionary* as administration through departments and subdivisions managed by sets of officials following an inflexible routine. Large organizations such as school systems usually become bureaucratic institutions.

The major characteristics—and also the limitations—of a bureaucracy include:

Fixed areas of jurisdiction.
Superior and subordinate positions arranged through a hierarchy of authority and responsibility.
Systematic and consistent approaches in organizing information.
Motivation is provided by compliance with rules.
System of jobs presupposing adequate job training.
Communication is from the top down.
Administrative rules and policies that are stable and difficult to change.
Administrators that perpetuate their jobs by defining and rationalizing their roles.
Decisions are rendered by leaders.
Primary emphasis is on work output.

Even Max Weber, the German sociologist responsible for the early formation of the bureaucratic model as the "ideal," expressed fear that the structure would breed organizational conservatism characterized by impersonal social relations, hierarchical authority, and the separation of policy-making and administrative functions (Weber, 1946). A large number of research studies have focused upon the problems of a bureaucracy. Some of the more significant findings are reported below:

- Recent critics such as Bennis (1968) have suggested that at the time it was developed, the bureaucratic format was well suited socially and economically. However, since social, management, and economic conditions have changed, there seems to be a need for revision. Bennis recommends that skilled and specialized training and coordination replace rank as the principle of bureaucratic differentiation.
- Burns and Stalker (1961), Thompson (1965), and Litwak (1961) also feel that bureaucracies create social-psychological climates not conducive to creativity, change, decision making, human relations, and consequent employee satisfaction and productivity.

Studies investigating bureaucracy found that it:

1. limits individual control over job activities;
2. provides minimal outlet for creative abilities, thus reinforcing passivity, paternalism, and dependence;
3. produces apathy among the work force, relatively high rates of turnover, absenteeism, malingering, and production restriction;
4. adheres strictly to a hierarchy of authority.

Organizational Structure in a Bureaucracy

Dr. Edward Stainbrook, professor emeritus at the University of Southern California School of Medicine, has written:

> The difficulty with bureaucracy is that they pyramid control so that employees who are at the final interface between the client and themselves, have already been defaced. They are being controlled anonymously and impersonally by the organization and so, of course as they have been defaced, they pass it on—they deface you. (Dean, 1979, p. 2L)

Unfortunately, there exists a basic incompatibility between the tasks to be performed and the organizational structure of a bureaucracy. The tasks generally require quick, individual responses to unpredictable problems. Since, however, the organizational structure imposes a strict hierarchy, divisions of labor, and separation between policy making and administration, it becomes very difficult to provide fast personal service (Hasenfeld & English, 1974). The conflict between trying to do an excellent job under bureaucratic restrictions is, for many, a major source of stress. Other findings include:

- The larger the number of layers in the hierarchy, the more stressful the situation is to employees. One study reported by Gmelch (1977) found that 83 percent of school staff experienced conflict distress when there were six to seven levels of authority between teachers and supervisors, as contrasted with 14 percent in an organization with only three levels between teachers and supervisors. Because of this stress, a large number of employees choose to leave the system (Sarason, Sarason, & Cowden, 1975). Within the past ten years, the rate of job turnover in large educational organizations appears to be growing rapidly.

- Paul Lawrence and Jay Lorsch of the Harvard Business School suggest that the style of management should be a function of the type of task to be carried out. Simple, predictable tasks with short time perspectives ought to be approached in a traditional bureaucratic manner. Conversely, tasks that are complex, dynamic, and unpredictable demand a more democratic or "human relations" approach. Either way, caution about imposing a managerial style should be exercised, since individual, cultural, and technological differences exist in all school organizations.

- Likert (1961) emphasized the need to adapt management practices to employee characteristics. He wrote, "The leadership and other processes of the organization must be such that each member will view the experience as supportive and one which builds and maintains his sense of personal worth and importance" (p. 103). Dubin, Homans, Mann, and Miller (1965), in their article on leadership and productivity, reviewing empirical evidence, concluded that no single best style of management exists. Instead, the researchers emphasized that the most successful supervisory style is one adapted to a particular organization and its internal and external environment.

- Perhaps the most salient example is offered by Vroom (1960; 1964), who found that employee participation in decision making increases motivation, performance, and job satisfaction except for authoritarian or highly dependent individuals (who are unaffected by participatory decision making).

Any organizational model must be based upon the individual characteristics of the employees, as well as the nature of the job. An authoritarian approach is necessary for a highly efficient army, especially since individuals who remain in the military tend toward the extremes of dependency or authoritarianism. In organizations that demand problem solving, creativity, and technological innovations, the converse approach is more effective. However, in both types of organizations one will always find personalities that require a more individual management style.

JOB SATISFACTION

Researchers have consistently found that people who are satisfied with their jobs are healthier and outlive those who are discontented. Decreased levels of cardiovascular disease, ulcers, and other stress-related problems were evident among satisfied workers. Contented employees report that they have found meaning and rewards in their work. Researchers have identified the following:

- A study investigating the factors most affecting job satisfaction in five Midwestern corporations was conducted by Weitzel, Pinto, Dawis, and Jury (1973). Their study involved a factor analysis of those variables most significant to job satisfaction. Of the 28 factors studied, the most significant factors in supervisor/subordinate interactions involved communication, feedback, competence, and participative decision making. Specifically, in rank order, the following factors prevailed:
  1. human relations of supervision;
  2. competence of supervisor;
  3. feedback from supervisors;
  4. openness of communication channels;
  5. recognition from superiors;
  6. participation in decision making.
- In another study, Locke (1976) found that the most important factors related to job satisfaction were:
  1. mentally challenging work;
  2. personally interesting work;
  3. rewards for performance consistent with *an individual's needs;*
  4. working conditions that are not physically demanding;
  5. a climate conducive to high self-esteem.
- Ruch, Hershauer, and Wright (1976) found that successful job performance was more often the cause of job satisfaction than vice versa.

- Social climate and support, both at work and at home, appear to be a variable of major importance to the psychological well-being and job satisfaction of workers. Maslach (1976) found that job burnout rates seem to be lower for those helping professionals who have access to formal or informal programs in which they can discuss problems and get advice and support.
- Caplan et al. (1975) found that two variables of subjective environmental stress—low support from the supervisor and low support from others at work—correlated significantly with job dissatisfaction and depression.

Job dissatisfaction can also be caused by disillusionment. In preparing for a job, most people have substantial preconceptions about the nature and depth of the work they are to do. It is not uncommon to hear a new teacher say, "I studied for years to get this job, and I'm not doing what I thought I'd be doing." Frequently our expectations are quite disparate from the reality of the actual job. In addition, it is common to hear, "I'm not adequately prepared to do this job." Our training institutions often instruct in two-dimensional models. They teach by reading and lecturing, with only a minimum of on-the-job training. Seldom, if ever, are the political, social, psychological, or physical job demands discussed. Adequate training is just as important as selecting a job where one's strengths and abilities can be effectively used.

JOB TURNOVER

We have witnessed in the past few years an alarming rate of turnover within high-stress occupations. School administrators, teachers, police, public health workers, and many others are leaving their jobs in unprecedented numbers. Anecdotal data from those leaving point toward job dissatisfaction, powerlessness over their work destiny, excessive demands at the work place, and work overload as major contributors to job mobility. Significant studies include the following:

- Over three decades, Wickert (1951), in a study of turnover and morale among female employees of a telephone company, found a significant difference between those who stayed and those who terminated. Those remaining felt they were making a contribution to the company, were able to make autonomous, job-related decisions, and were able to express their feelings.
- Ross and Zander (1957) found that *recognition* and *autonomy* were inversely related to turnover.

- Lee and Shepard (1972), sociological researchers from the University of Kentucky, have done comprehensive studies of voluntary turnover among helping professionals. They consider the causal variables of job turnover to be:
  1. extraorganizational (relationships with recipients of services, occupation trends);
  2. organizational (size, structure, role specificity, role conflict, atmosphere, rewards);
  3. group (supervisor/subordinate expectancies, cohesiveness, communication, and supervisory climate); and
  4. individual (job involvement, job satisfaction, role perception, performance).
- Herzberg, Mauser, Peterson, and Capwell (1957) did an extensive study on the relationships between job satisfaction, morale, and job tenure. They found high morale related to longer tenure in 33 out of 37 studies. A number of other studies support the same conclusion (Fournet, Distefano, & Pryer, 1966; Vroom, 1964; Dawis, Lofquist, & Weiss, 1968; Katzell, 1957; Tannenbaum, 1962; and Hulin, 1968).

In comparing the causes of job turnover vs. the causes of occupational stress (Chapter III), it is evident that the causes are similar. Conversely, high job satisfaction and low turnover are more representative of management utilizing a supportive/participative organizational model in which employee relationships are enhanced.

SUMMARY

Bureaucracy, job turnover, and job dissatisfaction are distinctly and directly related to occupational distress. Many individuals believe that bureaucracy exists only in public or governmental organizations. However, bureaucracy is much in evidence in any large profit or non-profit corporation. As expected, the larger the organization, and more bureaucratic and less personal the relationships, the higher the rate of job turnover, dissatisfaction, and burnout.

A sociological truism exists: "The longer an organization exists, the further it gets away from its original purpose." Organizations, whether providing services or products, were originally small, generally personal, and had a limited set of objectives.

Schools, for example, were established purely to educate children in reading, writing, and arithmetic. As they became larger and more complex, they began to assume a greater number of functions. Almost a century ago it was decided that the platoon system observed in Austria provided a good educational model. Classrooms were divided on the basis of grades. Publishing houses began to thrive as they packaged materials for each grade level. Soon educational objectives became complex and multifaceted. Bureaucracy became evident through the development of policies and rules. Today, education has become the largest industry in the United States. Schools are now social agencies that provide not only basic skills, but medical (immunizations, fluoride), social (desegregation, free lunch), psychological (counseling), aesthetic (art, music), and many other services.

CHAPTER V

Burnout of School Administrators

Educational administrators of the 1980s are beset by more change, conflict, and stress than in any single decade since schools came into being. More responsibilities and duties are crammed into the administrator's day than ever before. School superintendents have often been identified as highly susceptible to stress, but recent data suggest that middle managers are much more likely candidates for "management disease" than any other group (Gmelch, 1977). It is the manager caught between upper levels of management and subordinates who experiences the most distress.

Mintzberg (1973) pictured the nature of administrative work as follows: (1) Unrelenting pace—rushing through the mail, receiving phone calls, attending meetings, and having few breaks. The major reason for the relentless pace is the open-ended nature of the educational manager's job: there is always more work to be done. (2) Brevity, variety, and fragmentation—the typical manager has 36 written contacts daily, a maximum of 15 minutes of uninterrupted desk work, and a day fragmented by constant parent, teacher, student, and higher management requests. This continuous "gear shifting" dramatically challenges the manager's effectiveness. (3) Action and reaction that affect planning, thinking, and implementing.

According to Peterson (1978), principals average thirteen activities per hour, although the number can range from four to fifty. More than 85 percent of their time is spent on tasks of less than nine minutes duration, and 40 percent of their day is filled with activities initiated by others. Peterson said that frustration can develop if the principal feels controlled by the job rather than in control of it.

Job-related pressure is causing many school administrators to choose either a career change or early retirement. An official report on "The School Principal," mandated by the State of California in 1977, indicated that 25 percent of all current school administrators were expected to leave within the next five years, that many were leaving through early retirement, and that this premature departure was mainly caused by excessive stress (Legislative Analyst, 1977).

The National Association of Secondary School Principals (NASSP) found the average principal works 50 weeks a year, 56 hours a week including an average three evening meetings a week (Hendrickson, 1979). Scott Thomson, deputy executive director of NASSP said, "With the new demands of today and the older traditional demands, what you have is two full-time jobs rolled into one. But there's still only one person—the principal—to handle it all" (p. 25). It has been noted, in addition, that there are not enough assistants to help the principal. David Byrne, NASSP researcher, succinctly stated, "Most schools have more assistant football coaches than assistant principals" (p. 25). The previous assistance provided by teachers has dwindled due to collective bargaining contracts. NASSP reported that 40 percent of principals surveyed indicated they no longer experience fulfillment from their jobs (p. 25).

A *Newsweek* article on burnt-out principals (Seligmann & Huck, 1978) indicated: "In a recent survey of 1600 principals conducted by the University of Utah, one quarter said they intend to quit. . . . Worse yet, the very best principals are quitting at an even higher rate. At the beginning of the survey, researchers singled out sixty exceptional principals. A year later *one third* of this special group had resigned." Donald Thomson, superintendent of schools in Salt Lake City, lamented, "The really top principals are leaving the schools. They are going into better-paying jobs that offer more job satisfaction. There just isn't any way to keep them" (Hendrickson, 1979, p. 24).

Perhaps few other occupations have more extensive responsibility than a school administrator. The job requires working with more supervisors and recipients of services than in any other profession.* These include parents, school board members, advisory groups, state and federal bureaucrats, district administrators, teachers, and most importantly, students. A *Wall Street Journal* editorial ("Teacher Burnout," 1979a) stated,

---

* Appendix K includes a matrix listing 59 responsibilities that a principal must manage.

Deciding whether to suspend a bad student and commit work time to
a due-process hearing is but one of the principal's new duties. He is
now on the front line administering nearly every new program, rule
and law mandated by federal and state agencies and the courts. There
are detailed regulations for affirmative action on teacher recruitment,
special education, school-lunch programs and more. This used to be a
prestigious job, but many principals now feel they've become low-level
bureaucratic robots at the beck and call of legislators, parents and pressure groups. Thus, more are closing their doors on the hallway chaos,
or quitting. (p. 20)

Strong evidence supports the conclusion that as the principal goes,
so goes the school. If, in fact, the quality of school administrators has
a determining effect upon student performance, the loss of effective,
experienced leadership in our schools can be devastating. The *School
Effectiveness Study* (California State Department of Education, 1977,
p. 22) concluded that high-achieving schools were staffed by principals
having longer experience at these same schools. Teachers at these
schools reported that their administrators gave them individualized
support and guidance, while providing them with decision-making powers and influence in curriculum and school functioning. This concept
was substantiated in New York by a study which found that better quality of principal leadership was associated with higher student reading
achievement in low socioeconomic schools (New York State Office of
Education Performance Review, 1974, pp. 11–13).

A California task force headed by Assemblyman Dennis Mangers
concluded (Mangers, 1978) that principals are, in fact, the major
change agent in schools and have a direct influence on student performance.

CURRENT CONDITIONS OF ADMINISTRATORS

The traditional role of school administrators before 1970 included
working with parents, supervising staff, overseeing student discipline
and progress, managing the building, ordering supplies, and providing
general support to the school district central office. Most administrators found the role manageable and rewarding.

Since 1970, schools have become a hotbed of change and demands.
Within the past decade a host of new program adjustments have been
mandated: bilingual education, legal rights for handicapped students,
desegregation requirements, and collective bargaining for teachers, to
name but a few. New demands involving time, resources, paper work,

and community participation have besieged administrators. The energy required to resolve conflicts, meet with advisory groups, deal with new pressure groups, provide staff training, and disseminate information regarding mandated programs and new regulations is awesome. The need for more help in managing stress could not be greater. A 1978 report by the Association of California School Administrators concluded: "A number of forces are changing the role of the school site leader/administrator. As a result of these forces, many principals feel overwhelmed. They often feel also that their authority has diminished, and they feel they have been placed in impossible positions" (p. 1).

According to Vetter (1976), the school administrator is faced with demands from many quarters. The administrator must respond to pressures at the school level (from teachers, students, aides, support personnel), as well as to external demands from sources such as school board members, parents, superiors, teacher organizations, city officials, law enforcement officers, social workers, and citizens without children in school. Vetter concluded that the job of school administrator is a "killer," and that careful attention and assistance in reducing the pressure should be addressed.

The school administrator's job is not only highly responsible, but difficult and lonely. Surveys of administrators have found that the problems of being an administrator have increased, while the satisfaction has diminished. More is expected from schools today, but fewer resources are available to meet the demands. School administrators have acquired so many new responsibilities in the past ten years that they are now overextended.

THE PLIGHT OF THE MIDDLE MANAGER

Middle management can be considered the most frustrating position in organizational life (Albrecht, 1979). Demands from employees pull in one direction, while pressures from higher-level managers pull another way. Middle managers, eager to succeed and anxious to perform, feel responsible for pleasing both boss and employee. Many managers fail to notice their body's reaction to prolonged stress, so they routinely go about their business unaware of the physical drain.

Unfortunately, one of the unseen dangers of managerial stress is its cumulative nature. When chronic distress has accumulated over a period of years, the manager often suffers a substantial health breakdown. Many managers do not begin to feel the effects until they are 45–50 years old. The young manager does not think about having to pay the bill 20 or 25 years later for an unhealthy organizational life style. Seldom does one have good health one day and a severe breakdown the next. The manager's health collapse is a slow development of years of reaction to psychological distress. Ulcers, heart attacks, and strokes are infrequently precipitous; they develop over a period of time and send out many warnings. Cardiovascular disease now strikes occupants of high-stress jobs 13 years sooner on the average than their counterparts working at low-stress jobs (Albrecht, 1979).

ADMINISTRATIVE STRESSORS

In Chapter III, the major causes of job burnout were described as: Control Over One's Destiny; Communication/Feedback; Work Overload/Underload; Contact Overload; Role Conflict/Ambiguity; Training Deficits; and Personal Factors. The causes of stress cited by school administrators in a 1979 survey (Cedoline) were unmistakably related to the same causes of job burnout. In rank order, the following causes were identified by school administrators as the major stressors (generic descriptors shown in parentheses):

1. Lack of sufficient resources, e.g., supplies, fiscal aid, help with evaluation, personnel, inservice funding, and so forth (Control Over One's Destiny; Training Deficits).
2. Lack of support from superiors and the public (Communication/Feedback).
3. Quantity of work (Work Overload).
4. Paper work (Work Overload).
5. Collective bargaining (Communication/Feedback; Work Overload).
6. Lack of clear direction of role from school board and superintendent (Role Conflict/Ambiguity).
7. Federal and state laws (Control Over One's Destiny).
8. Lacking control of students, teachers, and schools (Control Over One's Destiny).
9. Responsibility for child's total needs and assumption of many parental roles (Work Overload; Contact Overload; Role Conflict/Ambiguity).
10. Parent and community relationships and pressures (Contact Overload).

The direct relationship is evident between causes of job burnout and the top stressors identified by school administrators. Although far from an exhaustive list, the following specific stressors when combined are chief causes of current administrative distress. Each identified stressor has been assigned to one of the seven major cause categories.

Control Over One's Destiny

Federal and State Control

Federal involvement in public education programs, particularly categorical programs, has increased by over five times in the past 15 years. Likewise, in California for example, this trend has resulted in a threefold increase in state control. As more financial support is given, more control is gained by federal and state agencies.

Local autonomy and decision making have also become restricted by the proliferation of state and federal laws. Many new laws have created a wider scope of responsibility for administrators. Concomitant with their passage are legal interpretation, new district policies, program implementation, time demands, and higher costs. During the late 1970s alone, major legal changes have occurred. Some of the most significant changes have been in these many areas: restrictions on discipline, student rights, suspension/expulsion, child abuse, immunization, collective bargaining, special education, curriculum restructuring, finance, desegregation, bilingual education, Title IX, due process, search and serve (handicapped), school improvement, fluoridation, miscellaneous surveys and assessments, student minimum competency requirements, breakfast programs, disadvantaged youth programs, Indian education, architectural barriers (handicapped), early childhood education, development of advisory councils, parent education and involvement, compensatory education, Indochinese education, affirmative action, data collection, emergency plans, summer school programs, and revised evaluation procedures ad absurdem. These considerable new demands made on school administrators often have ominous consequences; complying with each requirement has an effect upon school staff, students, parents, and related services. The overwhelming complexity of assimilating and implementing new legal mandates places enormous demands on school managers.

Invariably, legal interpretation is necessary in order to properly implement the legislative fiats. Many school managers have said, "You have to be a Washington lawyer to read and understand what must be done." Sometimes, different interpretations can be made of the same public law. Local policy development may be required to comply with legal mandates. If the next 15 years bring the same volume of legislative change, it will surely spell the end to quality education and local control.

Student Discipline

According to a Gallup Poll (1975), the number one problem in our schools is discipline. Not only have state and federal laws restricted the ways in which discipline may be administered in schools, but courts have also further complicated the problem of student control. The courts have issued awards against individuals for disciplinary actions that have abridged newly defined due process rights of students. Many administrators have avoided discipline measures in fear of legal suits. Whether disciplinary action is right or wrong in any individual case is not the question. The issue instead is maintaining adequate control at the local community level without the constant fear of outside reprisal.

Fiscal Difficulties

About three years after the 1977 landmark initiative known as Proposition 13, in California, our most populous state, the level of expenditures for education as a percentage of personal income ranked 44th among the fifty states (California School Boards Association, 1981). California expends only 4.7 percent of its total school budget on administrative salaries, as compared to the 5.2 percent national average (Olivero, 1979). This figure is approximately one third of that expended by industry for management costs. The old saying, "You get what you pay for," may be appropriate to the state of education in California. With rising inflation and further decreased revenues, the ability of school administrators to provide conscientious fiscal management is questionable. During the 1979–80 school year, the California State Department of Education allocated approximately $11 per student for elementary textbooks at one grade level, yet mandated the purchase of three at a publishers' cost of $18. In all states this same inflationary trend continues for other costs such as utilities, transportation, and paper.

As employees justifiably bargain for more equitable salaries, fiscal management becomes more and more difficult. Administrators are often caught between the public cry for unrealistic conservation and the practical realities of prudent money management. Today, the monetary reserves of school districts are at an all-time low—so low, in fact, that given unforeseen expenses, many districts could face bankruptcy.

As human and material resources diminish (e.g., teachers, aides, supplies, supervisory help), and responsibilities increase, the administrator's control of his or her own destiny is adversely affected.

Comparison to Private Schools

The public's condemnation of public schools often ignores the selectivity process not available to them. Private schools have an enormous advantage not available to public schools. An insidious selection process allows them to choose the students (or parents) they will accept. The public schools must take, with few exceptions, everyone who applies for admission. Private schools, on the other hand, can select on the basis of behavior, intellectual prowess, financial support, and parent involvement. In recent years private schools have been deluged with applications; those students not felt to be appropriate are simply not accepted. Similarly, discipline (punishment, suspension, exclusion) at public schools has been drastically restricted due to laws and court decisions. Private schools, because they are not publicly funded, can impose disciplinary actions not available to public schools. Student progress is unquestionably greater in private schools, where groupings and size can be controlled by selection of pupils and avoidance of mandates. These facts are frustrating to school administrators, who know their jobs are often controlled more by outside forces than by themselves.

Student Mobility

In recent years the typical American family has averaged a move every three to four years. Some schools experience mobility rates two to five times that average. As people move in and out of school communities, it becomes difficult to achieve stability. Opportunities to establish close and lasting relationships diminish, and the values within a community change as the population shifts. Administration of a sequentially consistent curriculum is extremely difficult when the needs of today's student population are found not to match tomorrow's enrollment. The morale of staff members at high-turnover schools is often significantly lower than that within schools of low student mobility. Unfortunately, transience among parents is reflected in their children's performance. Given an unstable school community, it becomes very difficult to control for curricula, community support, teacher frustration, paper work, and school resources. Consistent community support and involvement, perhaps more than any other outside factor, assist the school administration in providing an educational program that enhances student achievement. Without this stability, each day represents an unpredictable set of circumstances.

Job Stability

Turnover among principals in California recently has averaged approximately 17–18 percent each year (Legislative Analyst, 1977, p. 26). The rate of turnover for superintendents is approaching 30 percent. In one county, there was almost a 50 percent turnover among some 35 superintendents in a 12-month period. Job security for school administrators has become tenuous. Administrators must be constantly vigilant of the fact that their jobs are on the line. As the position of administrator becomes more complex and difficult to perform, the question of job security becomes more pressing. When security about one's job becomes questionable, paranoia increases and self-esteem diminishes. As stressors and self-doubt intensify, performance is affected. It is then that loss of job security looms as an ominous threat.

Inability to Transfer or Terminate Personnel

Control over employees is typically the major charge of managers in both industrial and public enterprise. If an administrator is to manage, sufficient authority is necessary. Unfortunately, school administrators have minimal authority in these matters. California has one of the strongest teacher tenure laws in the nation. A report by John Stull (1978), California State Senator, indicated that only one out of 18,050 teaching credential holders might, in a single year, be up for discipline or dismissal. This figure is 30 times lower than among lawyers (one out of 616), doctors (one out of 576), or other civil servants (one out of 628) (Olivero, 1979).

The maze of legal restrictions that inhibit necessary action against inadequate employees is frustrating, and for some administrators, distressing. The problem is twofold. Administrators need more training in preparing comprehensive evaluations, discipline, and/or terminations. Secondly, some modification of current tenure law needs to be considered. Interestingly, the Stull report pointed out that evidence of incompetence alone is not sufficient to remove an inadequate teacher. It has been estimated by both industry and government that in every job or profession studied, approximately two to five percent of the practitioners are truly incompetent. The data from the Stull report indicated that in the five years studied, an average of nine teachers were disciplined or dismissed (there are approximately 187,000 credentialed teachers in the state of California). One need not be a mathematician to conclude that a serious problem exists.

Proliferation of advisory councils. It is currently possible for a given school to have as many as nine advisory councils, depending upon the number of special or categorical programs available to students. The volume of paper work, number of meetings, degree of disagreement among concerned parties, and overall demands placed upon administrators are extensive. One example might be in the development of atlernative schools within the public school system. A study in Palo Alto found that the life expectancy of an alternative school was 18 months; the reason for its short life was due primarily to disagreement about the philosophy and values of various alternative approaches. Complete agreement among members of any group is unlikely. Reaching concurrence on a school's educational program for children is totally impossible.

Time management. On the job, administrators do not and cannot control all of the variables that affect use of their time. Emergencies become commonplace, and deadlines are imposed by local, state, and federal regulations alike. Parents, teachers, board members, and superiors have perhaps more opportunity to determine an administrator's time than the person him- or herself. If a typical day is preordained by outside determinants, control over one's time may be restricted to the point that distress sets in.

Communication/Feedback

Communication distance. The administrator's role has been likened to Sisyphus rolling his stone up a mountain. The loneliness and struggle lead to communication problems, as well as psychological distance from fellow employees. Opportunities to share similar concerns and work directly with fellow administrators are often limited. If the job involves 56 hours a week and an endless treadmill of unresolved concerns, the level of fulfillment declines. The altruistic idealism that once accompanied the job can degenerate into a struggle for survival.

Since relationships are transient, and time often militates against supportive friendships with colleagues, a feeling of isolation can occur. Isolation is increased by the contradiction between an individual's ideals and the demands of the job. Some provision for meaningful communication among professionals is an absolute necessity if support is to be provided. It is perhaps even more crucial in the field of education, considering that the ultimate goal is to increase knowledge through communication. If open communication is not fostered by and modeled within our schools, it is unrealistic to assume that it will be developed by other elements of society.

Collective bargaining. With the advent of collective bargaining, the educational profession has inherited a host of new problems. Additional aspects of supervision, a need for evaluation "by the book," and role redefinition have assumed importance. We now see polarization among parents, strife between teachers and administrators, and inevitable conflict.

Admittedly, there has always existed a need for better working conditions (e.g., better equipment, supplies, wages) for school employees. However, collective bargaining has only emphasized differences between teachers and administrators. It may be argued that unions are necessary for profit-oriented companies that can exploit employees in order to obtain larger profits. In education and other service professions, however, it is more important that all employees work together closely for the benefit of recipients. The only real profit or reward for professionals is the betterment of humanity. To create factions within various groups simply reinforces the Roman principle, "divide and conquer." The purpose of educators must not be divisiveness, but rather helpful cooperation.

Solutions must be obtained from within. Collective bargaining tends to relinquish local autonomy and control. A return to local resolution with earnest, honest, and representative membership can only strengthen the neighborhood educational community, instead of negating its force through the use of outside intervention.

What used to be a relatively close and comfortable relationship between administrators and teachers has now become somewhat like a dysfunctional family. Petty differences are magnified into grievances which not only consume time and energy, but create a barrier to face-to-face resolution of problems. The formalization (filing of complaints, review, mediation) of this process has created great distance between two important employee groups. Today, at a time when our schools are receiving the lowest level of public support, the public loses further esteem for school systems when they witness intramural feuding. The pressures relative to collective bargaining are taxing to administrators and teachers alike.

The need to administer collective bargaining agreements further distances principals from school staffs and creates additional stress. Strict adherence to the contract can create strained feelings when teachers must follow regulations more appropriate to a factory than to a profession. The inability of administrators to give personal attention to staff needs in deference to the provisions of a contract can be demoralizing. Collective bargaining affects the daily management of our schools. Whatever seems to have been gained is at least balanced by what has been lost—open communication, staff morale, public support, and local control.

Collective bargaining also has had a direct effect upon an administrator's ability to control his or her own destiny. Wagstaff (1973) says as outside groups and teachers gain power, administrators lose it, but there is no concomitant loss of responsibility. Administrators are still expected to develop and maintain good educational programs without the power to make the most creative use of their primary resources— teachers.

Lack of peer review. In almost all professions there exists a means of internal peer review. Policies and procedures are established by the members of the profession, and a review process is provided to assure maintenance of a high level of professionalism. Many researchers have verified the merits of such a system. Peer pressure is often much more effective than crisis intervention by a superior body. Peer review affords the individual an opportunity to gain support, guidance, and assistance from colleagues, as well as an opportunity to gain confidence and correct problems.

In addition to the benefits which devolve for individuals, professions need assurance that malpractice will not jeopardize their ethical image. It is fair to suggest that a small percentage (two to five percent) of school administrators are less than competent. The evaluation process, however, should serve as a first-level preventative resource and also allow for identified problems to be defined and corrected by peer action. The benefits of peer involvement cannot be overestimated as an initial corrective measure. If an individual is unwilling to participate in a review by peers it is then the responsibility of the organization to take appropriate action. Peer review as a means of personal/ professional improvement is one means by which school administrators could regain some measure of badly eroded public support.

Work Overload

Supervision/evaluation. In the past ten years we have all witnessed a proliferation of specialized services—bilingual education, gifted education, specialized curriculum aides, expanded special education for the handicapped, and so forth. Personnel needs have expanded, and administrators find themselves responsible for the supervision of an increasing number of employees. Such supervision demands time (which is not always available), plus knowledge and skills in a multitude of special areas.

The typical urban or suburban school principal is responsible for the direct supervision and evaluation of some 40–50 individuals. The typical industrial manager seldom is responsible for more than 12 employees. Management studies have consistently found that one person should not be required to supervise and evaluate more than 5–12 individuals; school administrators have responsibility for supervision and evaluation of four to ten times that number, involving many different work categories (Cedoline, 1980). These categories usually include teachers, aides, special program personnel (nurses, psychologists, speech therapists), secretaries, noon duty workers, custodians, and cafeteria workers.

"Paper mountaineering."   Since legislative and accountability requirements continue, an enormous number of forms and reports are necessary. The regulations are frequently complex and often contradictory or confusing. If a school provides categorical programs, an administrator would typically be held responsible for completing some three to ten planning or evaluation reports of varying complexity. The increased volume of paper work within the past decade has been extraordinary. It has been estimated that paper work has increased by 400–600 percent since 1970.

Decision making.   The average educator is called upon to make approximately 400 decisions a day. Since many of those decisions affect the lives of children, it is important that they be based upon good information and clear legal interpretation. School administrators may be held personally liable for the results of their actions.

In industry, decisions are generally focused upon products. In schools, daily decisions affect the lives of what parents cherish most— their children. The wrath of a disgruntled consumer is seldom as punishing as that of an irate parent. Most administrators, like parents, want to do what is best for the child; however, there is not always clear agreement about what is best. In making a decision, the school administrator must consider a number of alternatives with the knowledge that any of the possible options is certain to face some opposition.

Motivation for change. When the quantity and difficulty of work reaches an overload level, motivation for change is extinguished. During the bombings of London in World War II, the populace spent endless days living in shelters. Deluged with bombs, privation, and fear, it became instinctive for them to withdraw and try to survive. School administrators under great stress react similarly. They are not motivated to come up with new ideas or plans, because of the amount of work that would be required and the number of critical constraints to be overcome.

Motivation for change is proportional to the chance for successful implementation. As pressures soar, more time and energy are devoted to defensive reactions and less are available for quality improvement. The safe approach is to avoid change. It is easier to be a Monday morning quarterback or armchair critic than to take a risk.

Equal rights requirements. The federal government, in a sincere and just attempt to assure equal rights, has had a significant impact on school programs. Federal guidelines call for a full-scale reassessment of curriculum, program, and hiring procedures. Specific measures must be taken if federal standards have not been met. Texts must be carefully reviewed to assure non-biased content. Emphasis on equal opportunity for all must be assured. The intent is certainly valid and meritorious, but providing equity at all levels is not an overnight undertaking, and the mandatory changes require access to resources not easily available. Resistance to change is frequently encountered from staff, students, and parents alike.

Extra time requirements. School administrators are in one respect like obstetricians—always "on call." When a teacher has an emergency, a police officer arrests a student, a former employee needs a job reference, a power failure occurs, a representative is needed for county meetings, a fund-raising event is proposed, an accident occurs, child abuse is reported, the principal is usually the first to be contacted. Being a school administrator means being on call, with all the demands and resultant distress that the term implies.

Contact Overload

Contacts with people. There are few other occupations that require more contact with different types of people than school administration. Typically, the work day involves direct interaction with teachers, other staff members, students, parents, and people representing interests outside the school community. Such contacts include people with very disparate backgrounds and expectations. They may be cooperative or hostile, caring or apathetic, informed or ignorant, helpful or disruptive, responsible or negligent ad absurdem.

The typical administrator spends more than 80 percent of the work day in problem solving with students, school personnel, and community members. Activities are frequently interrupted by concerned or angry parents, demanding teachers, and distressed students. Since a school administrator's job is not limited to 8:00 A.M. to 5:00 P.M., evenings and weekends are often committed to talking with people who need assistance. Unless phone calls are ignored, accessibility cut off, and visibility lost, there is seldom respite from direct contact with people. In Chapter III, research was cited which clearly demonstrated that continual direct contact with people is a prominent cause of distress and job burnout. It is not surprising that school administrators are subject to excessive stress when over 80 percent of their time must be spent in direct contact with people.

Role Conflict/Ambiguity

Number and variety of expected roles.   The role of a school administrator includes being a social worker, politician, minister, police officer, doctor, parent, boss, sales representative, psychologist, and business manager. Each role elicits different behavior and emotions. Since each interaction with a parent, worker, and child requires a different approach, an administrator must react like a chameleon in order to accommodate and show respect for individual characteristics. Such changes can have a wearing effect. To switch rapidly and repeatedly from one role and behavior to another is stressful and exhausting.

Politics of education.   The school administrator is charged with being responsive to the values, philosophies, and priorities of the entire school community. This task is literally impossible to perform without compromising some personal integrity. The competing demands of different factions within the community create some degree of conflict at best, and sometimes erupt into an open power struggle.

The California Task Force (Mangers, 1978) described the phenomenon in its report:

> Accountability, parity, power and decentralization are all common terms surrounding schooling today. They have one thing in common. They have to do with the politics of education. Events of past years,

for example, civil rights and inflation, have placed schooling squarely and overtly in the political arena. It is one institution over which its various constituencies still feel they have some control.

Typically, educators have attempted to be apolitical when it comes to their own business. That is no longer possible. Each school principal must have at least a rudimentary understanding of how the political and school systems operate. The principal has to understand why things are as they are if leadership is to be exerted.

Legislatures, boards of education, administrators, employee organizations, parents and community members are vying for power in order to be able to participate in making decisions about schools. In this process, conflicting things may happen. For example, legislatures and state education agencies demand more community participation in local school decisions while the same entities prescribe how schools should function, thereby limiting the scope of local decision making. (pp. 60–61)

Mitchell (1972) said that a principal today is a person caught in the middle. The principal is supposed to speak for the school, teachers, pupils, and neighborhood, hoping to provide for everybody the elements of a good education. But at the same time, the principal is supposed to represent the school board and the central office of the local school system and enforce their policies. Mitchell summarized, "It is not always easy to harmonize the two functions" (p. 6).

Having to "wear too many hats" in an attempt to satisfy everyone's needs is an impossible task, yet one expected of any school administrator. The inevitable conflict results in at least some frustration on the part of all individuals involved. The depth and intensity of the problem may vary from situation to situation, but it is omnipresent and a real source of distress.

Societal changes.   More than 50 percent of the mothers of school children are working, and 65 percent are expecting to be employed in less than five years. The divorce rate is at an all-time national high. Vandalism and crime are rampant (over $600 million is spent annually in repairing vandalism damage to schools in the U.S.). The control of parents over their children has been challenged by emancipation legislation. Many families are on the brink of economic disaster. Alcohol and drug addiction are common among young adults. Communities are plagued by rapid change and lack of a stable identity. Children and parents alike are faced with a complex new world which is often difficult to understand and assimilate. Most of these problems are the product of a society vexed with constant change. For better or worse, our schools reflect our society, and the manifestations are sometimes not appealing.

Administrators, often conservative individuals who bear traditional values, sometimes find it difficult to accommodate to changes and diversity within their respective communities. Stressors such as more discipline problems with limited alternatives for intervention, decreased availability of parents, vandalism and crime, diminished community involvement, less family stability, and shrinking evidence of support are coupled with increasing expectations that the school will serve as a surrogate for the family in such areas as nutrition, drug abuse, and sex education. Combined with other stress factors, the result is all too often the traumatic response known as burnout.

Individual Factors

An area which has received limited attention by researchers is the relationship between personal factors and occupational stress. Although supportive data is miniscule, there is evidence that the personal characteristics of individuals have some decided effect upon job performance and vulnerability to job stress. The following is only a superficial review of major personal characteristics.

Age/Professional experience.   Younger school administrators begin their careers filled with enthusiasm and idealism. As time passes, some begin to become disillusioned by the incongruity of what should be (ideal) with what is (real). Distress is cumulative and consequently begins to have a more noticeable affect between the age of 40–55. Older managers become disillusioned not only with their work but with their lot in life. Some people are distressed by their age and level of success. The phenomenon of middle-aged crisis needs further scientific investigation, but could be a factor in job dissatisfaction.

Family.   Most administrators are also parents. As children progress through the normal developmental stages, various problems are inevitable. If the managers work long hours committing evenings to the job, it is probable that family problems will result. Whatever the cause of such problems, they generate stress in the worker. According to a highly predictable health stress survey (Holmes & Rahe, 1967), the most significant stressors involve trauma within the immediate family.

Health.   Whether health problems are a cause of, or result from, occupational stress, the loss of productivity can be substantial. The body warns of impending problems and demands proper care for optimum functioning. Health problems, as noted earlier, are frequently associated with high stress jobs. Again, because of the cumulative effect of distress, health problems do not become visible until later in one's career.

Individual background.   If a person grows up in a stressful environment, there is usually one of two major outcomes—either the individual learns effective means of dealing with stress, or he or she succumbs to the pressure. In recent years physiological stress reactions have been measured through the use of sensitive electronic monitoring devices. First, physiological processes were measured to obtain baseline data. Then a stress test was administered. Typically, the person was asked to count backwards from 1,000 by 3s. To add additional stress, the individual might have been told that the last applicant completed the test in 12 minutes. All subjects elicited physiological stress reactions. More important, however, was how the person recovered from the stress. If the subject recovered quickly, it generally meant that he or she had developed the ability to handle recurring stress without becoming immobilized for periods of time.

An individual's day-to-day experiences, then, offer opportunities to learn stress-relief techniques. With the advent of stress monitoring devices, it has also been shown that people can be taught stress-inoculation skills.

Sex differences.   There are not enough data on the effect of administrative stress on women to suggest clear-cut sex differences. Women have only recently come to occupy larger numbers of higher-level school management positions. According to some reports, women have experienced significantly greater stress in communication/feedback areas where they are often excluded from male conversations or activities. Women have also reported more resentment and isolation from male co-workers. Role conflicts have also been mentioned as a potential stressor for women, who are often responsible homemakers as well as part of a management team. A great deal more research data will be necessary before any conclusions can be made.

On a somewhat different tangent, sexuality in relationship to work has been informally reported. Some school administrators have suggested that when work overload reaches exorbitant proportions, sexual desire is stifled. This is a sensitive issue, which is conspicuous in its absence from the research literature.

Use of alcohol or drugs.   The use of alcohol or drugs can have a devastating effect upon an employee's work performance. Individual differences might determine whether the use of drugs is a cause or an effect of occupational stress. Highly dependent or authoritarian personalities reportedly tend toward alcohol or drug use; however, the use of drugs is limited to no single personality type. In most industries, significant responsibility for the remediation of such problems is assumed by the company. Because of the assumed potential danger to students, schools have often moved to dismiss staff members who abuse the use of alcohol or drugs. A more responsible approach might be to relieve the individual from contact with children and arrange for necessary treatment.

Personal crisis or financial difficulty.   During times of personal crisis or financial difficulty, it is unlikely that an employee can give full and undivided attention to the job. Negative circumstances are likely to be defeating and emotionally draining. Again, individual differences dictate one's response. Under adverse conditions, some managers get so involved in their work that they distract themselves from their problems. Others become so encapsulated in their personal difficulties that they ignore work. Very little research is available to provide discriminating diagnoses of the reactions of different individuals.

Value system.   Each individual enters the world of work with a unique set of values. Those people who value responsible and honorable work assignments are often the most productive and successful. Those who seek employment for prestige or salary are sometimes less productive. Unfortunately, the research data strongly points toward job burnout for those employees who are the most conscientious, loyal, and responsible. These individuals have difficulty saying no and respond immediately to supervisory demands or recipient needs. An organization, in order to not lose its most valuable employees, must take preventative and remedial action to nourish and protect these vulnerable workers.

Training Deficits

Lack of Preparation for Current Problems

The contemporary role of the school administrator calls for expertise as: creator, coordinator, implementor, communicator, negotiator, problem solver, motivator, placator, evaluator, catalyst, counselor, organizer, researcher, supervisor, lawyer, politician, accountant, discipline agent, personnel manager, writer, public relations specialist, parent surrogate, health and safety specialist, instructor, and most importantly, student. The Association of California School Administrators (1978), in "Changing Role of the Principal," has compiled a 67-page job description of the principal's duties. The publication documents the fact that many administrators are no longer adequately prepared to undertake today's expanded role.

As mentioned earlier in this chapter, Assemblyman Dennis Mangers completed a major study of school administrators. The report was presented to the California Assembly in 1978 with the specific recommendation that more training and preparation be provided for school administrators. The findings of the task force basically concluded that principals are the major change agent and have a direct effect upon student performance. The task force declared that adequate preparation and ongoing training are an absolute necessity. To maintain school leadership, the principal must be well informed and adequately prepared for a new and expanding role. The Mangers report was very clear on this issue. It stated,

> The principal will demonstrate a willingness to keep abreast of current developments in the field through a stated plan of self-development, which includes reading, participation in inservice activities, conference attendance, visitations and/or other professional development activities. (p. 64)

McNally (1975) aptly commented:

> Any modern production-for-profit enterprise that failed to provide for the retraining of workers to cope with changing technology and product design would soon go out of business. Yet, well-conceived provisions for the inservice development of principals are rare in school systems in this country. (p. 25)

It is difficult to understand the current lack of state-funded administrative training. Training for administrators in at least the following areas is crucial for protection against burnout: renewed management and leadership skills, self-awareness, facilitation of group processes, public relations, decision making, stress management training, instructional skills, employee motivation and evaluation, legal updates, negotiation and collective bargaining, and time management.

It is very important for administrators to identify areas of professional need and to contract in their evaluation goals for their accomplishment. More importantly, time and some form of assistance must be provided to make the process effective and meaningful. There is probably no other single time-off procedure that reaps higher dividends. As paid and volunteer aides are available for teachers, there needs to be a similar system available to administrators to free them for renewal activities. Assistance may come from retired personnel, prospective administrative candidates, or temporary interns. The expense of aides or substitutes can be cost-effective if adequately planned. If schools are charged with educating, the leaders of our schools must first be educated.

SUMMARY

We have begun to see an acceleration in an unfortunate and expensive trend: the loss of highly trained and experienced school administrators to a phenomenon identified as "job burnout." Complex demands upon administrators are triggering an increasing number of resignations, job changes, and premature retirements.

Growing pressure from every quarter—school boards, employee organizations, parents, courts, federal and state bureaucracies, and legislative bodies—dramatically affects the job efficiency and effectiveness of school administrators. At this time of crisis within our schools, we cannot afford to lose highly trained and experienced administrators.

There is an urgent need for the public to gain awareness of causes and of current conditions. Public support and assistance are necessary to remediate existing conditions and prevent further disruption among our troubled educational leaders. Although the process of decay has started, our school system continues to survive on the strength of its solid (though threatened) foundations.

There is a ray of light—relief is possible if public awareness is forthcoming. If sincere efforts by the educational community can be sustained and nourished, we may be able to control the level of administrative burnout. Board and community members must become aware of the real, imminent, and severe plight of their managers. Enlightened school administrators, recognizing the scope and nature of the problem, can serve to educate others, provide internal support to troubled colleagues, and cooperate in the search for effective means to prevent and cure occupational distress.

CHAPTER VI

Teacher Burnout

> "Many teachers feel they were responsible for the invention of the microwave—so they could correct papers, cook, and watch the evening news simultaneously."

Statistical data indicate that teachers are abandoning the profession in increasing numbers. Many are finding jobs in private industry, others are seeking early retirement, and still others are simply dropping out. Thousands of teachers have laid down their pointers and chalk largely because of decreased funding, limited personal control over their teaching, and lack of societal commitment. One national survey by the National Education Association (McGuire, 1979) indicated that one-third of all teachers surveyed wished they could be doing something else.

One important factor which contributes to this trend is teacher burnout. Burnout is a more serious problem to the profession than job change or early retirement because it renders a teacher unable to cope, although he or she remains in the classroom. The loss of energy and enthusiasm to teach is strong evidence of teacher burnout. According to Truch (1980), teacher distress costs at least $3.5 billion annually through absenteeism, turnover, poor performance, and waste. According to one study (Kyriacou & Sutcliffe, 1975) one-quarter of all teachers feel burned out at any given time.

Sally Reed of *Instructor* magazine expressed the belief that victims of burnout "will either leave the profession after years of training and dedication, or remain in the classroom immobilized by inertia, no longer caring." Teacher burnout is not a new phenomenon, but it has increased to epidemic levels in the past five years.

The pride felt by educators—at one time among the highest in the professions—is beginning to dwindle. Informal surveys have found that most teachers like to teach and would prefer not to leave, but they feel their previous level of satisfaction has dramatically diminished. Many talk of constant frustration, disillusionment, diminished community support, and fewer rewards. Schools of education have announced a 20 percent drop in teacher-training applicants. The NEA reported that in 1961, about 28 percent of America's teachers had 20 or more years' experience. Using the same survey in 1976, it was found that this figure had decreased to 14 percent. More frightening was that 40 percent of those teachers presently working planned to leave before reaching the normal retirement age.

TEACHER DISTRESS

The incidence of distress among both beginning and experienced teachers is remarkably high. The subject of teacher anxiety has received considerable attention since early in this century. In 1933 during the Great Depression, Hicks found an incidence of 28 percent of teachers having significant nervous conditions. That same year, Peck found 33 percent of women teachers surveyed had nervous symptoms. In 1938, the NEA reported that 37.5 percent of a nationwide sample of over 5,000 teachers expressed serious worry and nervousness. In 1951, NEA did a similar study and found 43 percent of the 2,000 teachers sampled indicated "considerable strain and tension." In 1976 another NEA survey found that 78 percent of the teachers reported moderate to considerable levels of stress. The continuing rise in the incidence of moderate to severe stress is alarming.

Willard McGuire (1979), president of NEA, expressed the belief that, "Stress is leading to teacher burnout and the problems threaten to reach hurricane force if it isn't checked soon" (p. 5). A 1979 NEA resolution ("Stress on Teachers," 1979) stated:

> The National Education Association believes that the dynamics of our society and increased public demands on education have produced adverse and stressful classroom and school conditions. These conditions have led to increased emotional and physical disabilities among teachers and other school personnel.
>
> The Association urges its local affiliates, in cooperation with local school authorities, to develop stress management programs that will facilitate the recognition, prevention, and treatment of stress-related problems.
>
> The Association further urges that the harmful effects of stress on teachers and other school personnel *be recognized,* and it demands

procedures that will ensure confidentiality and treatment without personal jeopardy. (p. 36)

The most common initial stress symptoms reported by teachers are irritability, depression, sleeping problems, headaches, stomach disorders, and shortness of breath. Many fail to recognize these budding problems as work-related. Consequently, teachers do not ask for help or share their problems with others. Although much mental energy is given to these problems, few are brought out in the open. Many teachers are embarrassed to share their difficulties with fellow workers. Instead, they often (mistakenly) shrink from seeking the assistance of others because they perceive that they should be extending rather than receiving help.

Teachers are reinforced for unselfish behavior. Like many other professionals, teachers feel they should be able to handle their own stress. Many expect to live up to an ideal or storybook figure who is always able to overcome adversity. Unfortunately, the burnout rate does not reflect the viability of these superhuman expectations.

CAUSES OF TEACHER DISTRESS

It is not surprising that the specific causes of teacher burnout are the same as or similar to those of administrative burnout. It logically follows that if schools represent a somewhat bureaucratic hierarchy, stress would be channeled down through the ranks. Although individual researchers report slightly different specific causes, nearly everyone can be categorized under the seven major causes of job distress. The multitude of causes include public pressure, legislative proliferation, extremes of assignment (ranging from no avenues for change to involuntary placement in less desirable settings), violence, limited feedback and support, student behavior, budgetary reversals, media assault, and collective bargaining.

Researchers have consistently found a strong relationship between job satisfaction and teacher mental health (Gechman & Wiener, 1975; Kasl, 1973). If teachers find positive satisfaction and success in their work, they will better resist stress. Unfortunately, we are now in an era of limited job satisfaction in which the mental anxiety of teachers is at an all-time high. A study by Sparks (1979) found the following:

- Forty-six percent of the teachers surveyed were dissatisfied with their job as a whole, and said if they were to do it over again they would not choose teaching as a career.

- Over 54 percent said they would probably not stay in teaching until retirement, and would likely change careers in five years.
- Seventy percent said they frequently or always left school physically or emotionally exhausted.
- Thirty-six percent said work at school affected their home life.
- Ninety-one percent said they had little or no influence on curricula or policy decisions.
- Only 23 percent said they had high-quality relationships with their administrator.
- Some 73 percent said they felt pulled in different directions by expectations of students, parents, and administration.
- High-level dissatisfaction was expressed regarding involvement in decision making and communicating with administration.

Mohrman, Cooke, and Mohrman (1978) found clear evidence that teacher satisfaction was not just related to the degree to which they participated, but also to the type of involvement; teacher satisfaction was strongly related to involvement in "technical decisions" (e.g., tests, learning problems, instructional activities) or areas that directly affect teachers. No significant relationship was found between management-type decisions and teacher satisfaction. The issue for teachers may not be one of participation in managerial decisions (hiring, faculty assignments, budget planning), but rather in decisions affecting instruction. Truch (1980) reported the results of a study involving 800 teachers in 21 school systems. Teachers were found to be most satisfied with areas that they could control (classroom activities), and least satisfied with areas of very little control (societal attitudes) that affected their performance.

Hundreds of studies have focused on the causes of teacher stress. One of these (Coates & Thoresen, 1974) was a comprehensive review of teacher anxiety. It found that experienced teachers reported that time demands, difficulties with pupils, large class enrollments, financial constraints, and lack of educational resources were the major sources of teacher stress.

Instructor magazine ("Teacher Burnout," 1979b) reported that teachers in Chicago had rated 35 school-related situations on an inventory of teacher stress. Those causing the most stress were involuntary transfers, disruptive students, threats of personal injury, assault on a colleague, and verbal abuse. The least stressful events were teaching curricula and meeting with parents.

Mattox (1974) investigated the reasons why teachers quit their jobs. He found no single factor that influenced teachers to leave the profession, but he did find groups of factors that led to stress and consequent departure. Some of the major causes of tenured teachers' leaving were long hours, inadequate salary, lack of advancement, too many evening responsibilities, lack of administrative support and backing on decisions, submission of state reports, oversized classes, and discipline problems. The study revealed a strong implication that if stressors were not controlled, many teachers would be motivated to find another occupation with less degree of stress.

Pratt (1978) analyzed the perceived stress of 124 primary school teachers and found that the level of financial deprivation in students' home backgrounds was positively and highly significantly related to perceived stress of teachers. He also found that teacher stress increased with the age of children taught. In addition, a significant correlation was found between the amount of teacher stress recorded and illness of teachers measured by a general health questionnaire.

In 1979 the Tacoma, Washington, school system conducted a survey of working conditions among its employees ("Teacher Burnout," 1979c) and found the most significant stressors were involuntary transfer (most stressful), notification of unsatisfactory performance, assault upon a colleague, managing disruptive children, and disagreement with a supervisor. The study found that Tacoma was losing some of its best teachers. The report included the appalling finding that one-quarter of the teachers had been physically assaulted, and three-quarters reported having been verbally abused (p. 7).

Control Over One's Destiny

Involuntary Reassignment

With the advent of decreased enrollments, financial difficulties, and court-imposed busing and programs, teachers are leaving their jobs at record rates. As a result of court-ordered racial balance decisions, literally thousands of teachers quit in both Los Angeles and New York rather than accept involuntary transfer. When the New York City Board of Education attempted to rehire 9000 furloughed teachers (1977–78), fewer than *one out of three* returned ("Teacher Burnout," 1979b, p. 57).

Involuntary reassignment has been noted as a major cause of teacher distress. Teachers, like other professionals, resist changes—particularly those that involve the unknown, and especially when changes suggest demotion or abandonment. Unfortunately, reassignments, although necessary, are usually made without direct communication with those affected.

Discipline/Behavioral Control

NEA has cited a number of reasons for teacher burnout, the most important of which is a pervasive sense that teachers have lost effective control of their classrooms. In the past, 20 percent of the children demanded 80 percent of the teacher's time. Today teachers report that these problem children are even more difficult to control. In his study of perceived stress among teachers, Pratt (1978) found that the home background of the students is a major and pervasive influence in creating stress. He discovered marked increases in reported stress among teachers of children from financially deprived homes.

Inner city schools that experience severe behavioral problems among their students almost certainly suffer huge teacher turnover. Even extra pay, referred to by some as "combat pay," is not attracting skilled teachers. Physical assaults are becoming commonplace even at the elementary level. Two large cities, Los Angeles and New York, are severely understaffed with special teachers to work with behavior and learning-problem children. Both have taken out large ads and are completing a national search.

The rise of physical violence in schools reflects other national problems. In 1975 alone, over 66,000 attacks on teachers were recorded in U.S. public schools. In 1979 there were an estimated 110,000 physical assaults on teachers, or assaults on one out of every twenty teachers (McGuire, 1979, p. 5). According to Alfred Bloch of the department of psychiatry at U.C.L.A., many inner city teachers live in constant fear of violence and develop "combat neurosis" ("Teacher Burnout," 1979b). The symptoms include unnecessary fears, shell-shock reactions, insomnia, high blood pressure, exhaustion, and sometimes collapse. Similar symptoms are found in advanced degrees of job burnout.

Salary

Teachers have limited control over their livelihood. A few years ago a friend of the author decided to go back to school and become a teacher. He enjoyed children, his father had been a school board member, and he always had a desire to teach. He continued working full-time at a grocery store while attending college. After five years he finished his credential program and received several teaching offers. He was filled with consternation when he reported, "I've made up my mind. I can't take a teaching job. With a wife and baby, I just can't afford to take a $9,000 a year cut in salary from my job as a grocery clerk. Besides, our insurance and benefits are a lot better with the clerks' union." Besides state and local school boards' maintenance of strong conservative control over salaries, two-digit inflation has further deteriorated the paychecks of teachers. In addition, excellent performance is not rewarded with extra incentives. Most teachers are humble and selfless, yet the reality of sharing in the "American dream" is a reality which is both sought and believed.

Decision Making

Teachers must be able to find satisfaction and motivation through some degree of autonomy and control. Satisfied teachers are those who participate in major classroom and curriculum decisions. They enjoy the opportunity to support their schools, parents, and students.

If all major decisions are left to various pressure groups or administrators, teachers begin to feel helpless about their control, particularly over matters of curriculum which they must implement. There is ample documentation to support the view that teacher participation in decision making has desirable consequences. Studies done in industry dating from the famous Western Electric Studies at Hawthorne, Illinois, to many later studies (e.g., Vroom, 1960) support the positive effect of employee involvement. Teachers who report that they participate in decision making consistently also report enthusiasm about their school system. Participation has desirable consequences for morale, productivity, and job satisfaction. Decisions that affect teachers without their involvement limit their feelings of control in their classrooms.

Supervision/Evaluation

Unsatisfactory evaluation and disagreement with one's supervisor have been cited as significant teacher stressors.

Conflicts between teachers and administrators have been aggravated by the increased responsibilities and demands already cited. Since the advent of collective bargaining, teachers and administrators have polarized into "labor" and "management" identities. As relationships become strained, stressors increase; evaluation becomes more formal and impersonal; fear increases while trust evaporates. Polarization and heightened demands also tend to intensify the feeling among teachers of less control over their job.

Teacher evaluations tend to focus on two major variables—personal characteristics and student achievement. Personal variables include such factors as organization, neatness, classroom management, use of materials, enthusiasm, cooperation, participation in school activities, and meeting deadlines.

The second, more accountable, measure is student progress. Achievement of pupils is usually based on standardized tests, which do not always reflect the school district and teacher's curricula. Teachers are also cognizant that learning is not always under the direct control of schools. These misgivings and fears cause teachers to promise less when they develop their annual objectives, in order to assure successful accomplishment of projected student growth. A conflict exists between teachers' taking responsibility for reaching certain levels of achievement, and their lack of authority and control over classroom activities and conditions. The statement of former Vice-President Walter Mondale (1979) is appropriate, "Get educated, caring people in the classroom; then let them alone and let them work."

Student Rights

Many good-minded people in the 1960s decided that there needed to be a large-scale expansion of student rights, particularly the right of due process. This movement was led by the American Civil Liberties Union (ACLU) as an attempt to curtail what was seen as repressive school control tactics. A rash of court decisions as well as state and federal laws were rendered. One decision established that a student cannot be suspended from school without the opportunity to respond to charges. Another decision required signed parental permission before any corporal punishment could be administered. Courts also made personally liable those who did not provide adequate due process or who abridged any student's rights. Although the intent is commendable, the rulings have caused great consternation among the educators who have had to implement them daily in the field.

Many teachers, unsure of their own rights, now impose discipline less forcefully and with caution. Faced with the real or implied threat of legal action, teachers have become timid because of their perceived lack of authority. It is little wonder that a Gallup Poll (1975) concluded that discipline is the number one problem in America's schools.

(Other factors such as state and federal control, fiscal difficulties, private schools, and student mobility are also directly related to teachers' control over their destiny. Consult Chapter V for a discussion of these subjects.)

Communication/Feedback

Limited Feedback

More than ever before, feedback to teachers has been limited to (1) the time available for access to administrators/fellow teachers, and (2) the evaluation process. The availability of school administrators for informal discussions has become limited in the past decade (see Chapter V). Personnel evaluation has become a highly structured process often not accommodating periodic feedback or informal meetings. As principals become overwhelmed, the quality and quantity of guidance and feedback which they can furnish suffer. Consequently, teachers seek and come to rely on feedback from other sources.

As public involvement, support, and respect decline, positive feedback from those sources diminishes. Teachers must often work without easy access to information that would allow them to monitor their performance. Little positive reinforcement is given to most teachers, but negative feedback is immediately forthcoming whenever an error is made or a disagreement arises. A steady flow of only negative response is counter-productive and highly distressful. Feedback of an honest and constructive nature is the sustenance of success.

(Other communication/feedback factors mentioned in Chapter V are also related to teacher stressors.)

Work Overload and Contact Overload

Class Size

The subject of class size has been one of the most long-standing and controversial issues in education. School trustees have argued that class sizes of up to 35 students are manageable, and they have sometimes cut costs by increasing class size. Studies have been cited by school boards and administrators to show that class size is not a significant factor in school achievement. Teachers, on the other hand, have claimed that large classes of heterogeneous students are indeed less manageable, and they also have cited supportive research data.

Maslach and Pines (1977) found that the quality of professional interaction is greatly affected by the number of people for whom the worker is providing care. As numbers increase, cognitive, sensory, and emotional overload results. When the professional has fewer people to worry about, he or she can provide more and better attention to each individual. Several studies have shown that teachers with small classes provide more encouragement, attention, and intimacy. Teachers of larger classes devote significantly more time to control and discipline, and display fewer positive behaviors.

Glass and Smith (1979a,b) have completed the most exhaustive and extensive study of class size thus far. Their research included 80 different controlled studies involving more than 900,000 pupils. Classes ranged from a few students participating in tutorial activities to classrooms with more than 60 students. Their conclusions follow:

- School subject matter made little difference, but both positive and negative effects were slightly greater in secondary than in elementary schools.
- A good teacher in a large class may produce better results than a mediocre teacher in a smaller class.
- Achievement levels increase significantly in classes with fewer than 20 children per teacher, but remain relatively the same whether there are 30, 40, 50 or over 60 children in the class.
- Controlling for teacher and other variables, pupils in a class of 15 or less will achieve significantly more than those in a class of 30.
- Reducing class size from 30 to 25 will bring no significant or noticeable change in student achievement.

The findings of Glass and Smith may actually be reassuring to school boards, teachers, and administrators alike. It may not be feasible to limit class size to one teacher for every 15–20 children, but it may be possible to make other changes. Glass and Smith suggest that school districts might make greater use of teacher aides, paraprofessionals, and parent volunteers in order to approximate optimal learning ratios.

In a similar vein, the author polled housewives, factory workers, and middle managers from private industry to determine their willingness to take responsibility for 30–35 children, six hours a day, for 36 weeks of the year. The results found more than 90 percent unwilling to assume this awesome responsibility. Frequent comments were, "That's why I send them to school"; "Teachers are trained to do that"; "I have enough trouble with ten adults"; or "Is this a joke?"

Student Population Changes

Within the past ten years, particularly in California, Florida, and Texas, there has been a substantial immigration of non-English-speaking students. This addition of Cuban, Mexican, Vietnamese, and other

ethnic groups has often taken place without additional teaching resources. Concomitant with the arrival of these special-needs children
has been a declining enrollment due to diminished birth rate and expansion of private schools. Classroom size, on the other hand, has not
generally changed. Instead, decreased revenues have caused teacher
layoffs and elimination of some services. These factors place a classroom teacher in a situation with extremes of student performance
levels. In a typical graded classroom of 32 students, there can be as
many as six to eight different grade levels of performance. For example, a fourth-grade class may easily contain non-English and En-
glish-speaking students with pre-primer (kindergarten or less) reading
levels, as well as children with seventh- and eighth-grade skills.
Grouping and instruction under these overload circumstances are
both challenging and difficult. The concept of the one-room school-
house continues to exist in a typical classroom in any given inner city
school system.

(Other work overload and contact overload factors mentioned for
administrators in Chapter V are also teacher stressors.)

Role Conflict

Mass Education vs. Individualized Instruction

Public schools have traditionally been organized for mass education. The democratic goal of free public education includes meeting
the needs of a diverse, heterogeneous group of students, each entering
at a different intellectual, psychological, and social level. Curricula
are designed to instruct the majority of students. Consequently, general lesson plans to accommodate large groups of students within uni-
form schedules often neglect individual differences.

Teachers recognize the discrepancy between the necessity of dealing with total classes and the ideal of individual instruction. Unfortunately, youngsters of all achievement levels must fit into the general scheme of a mass educational program. The most desirable
situation would be to provide for each student, where teachers fit the
program to the child and not vice versa. Optimally, equal time and
concern should be insured for each youngster. Student success would
then be defined by the child's entering level, motivation, skills, abilities, and personality. Pragmatically, however, a teacher with 30–35
children cannot provide the total equality of an individualized approach.

Teachers know that they should provide an excellent educational program for all assigned students. At an emotional level, however, teachers also know that it is nearly impossible. This conflict is extremely frustrating. Most teachers consistently make adjustments for the special needs of children. Some teachers have four or five different groups for each of several subjects. Time is invested in planning, record keeping, evaluating, and monitoring the progress of each child. Guilt accumulates as teachers admit to themselves that they should be doing more for some children. Frustration is accelerated as parents demand greater accountability. Commitment to the ideal of individual development in a context of mass education creates a mutual sense of inadequacy and dissatisfaction between teachers and the educational system.

Conflicting Values

A great many social and cultural demands are placed upon the school system. Industry demands that schools teach children about careers and jobs; some parents demand emphasis upon basic skills, while others demand enrichment and social skills; many civic groups demand citizenship and values training, while others seek sex education or awareness among school personnel of child abuse; legislators demand equal rights, due process, and holistic education; church groups demand moral education and time for religious activities; agnostic groups demand that schools eliminate anything that speaks of God; minorities demand more representative hiring, cultural awareness, and multilingual education; and assorted interest groups lobby for things such as metric mathematics or evolutionary theories.

Although each demand may be important, the ability of school systems to provide is finite. It becomes less and less possible for schools to teach everything to everybody. As demands increase, teachers become overwhelmed with the myriad of unranked priorities. As schools become the focal point of social change, they fall prey to bewilderment and frustration. It is clear that schools as they are currently organized cannot provide a cure-all for all the demands of society.

(Other role conflict/ambiguity factors discussed for administrators in Chapter V are also teacher stressors.)

Individual Factors

Personality Characteristics

Most individuals who have chosen teaching as a profession are disposed by their personalities to specific attitudes and aptitudes.

Those who teach are generally more dedicated to their work than most employees in industry. They enjoy working with children and have a sincere desire to help others. Prospective teachers have themselves attended school for many years and have a clear picture of the potential difficulties of the classroom; yet they choose their profession out of an unselfish desire to instruct and guide students. Almost all are aware of the low salaries and sometimes difficult working conditions in education. The personality characteristics of altruism, sincere caring, and idealism—when met by lack of feedback, limited appreciation, public apathy, and day-to-day stress—make teachers vulnerable candidates for occupational distress.

Training Deficits

Preparation and Self-Renewal

Beginning teachers may experience occupational stress as a result of deficits in their preservice preparation. Often their training has created unrealistic expectations that lead to substantial disillusionment and frustration. Teachers frequently find that their educational preparation has not been sufficient for the actual demands of the job. Today, more than in any other time in educational history, teachers need comprehensive training in order to perform effectively what has become an extremely complicated job.

Self-renewal is important for all teachers in order for them to be able to provide the spectrum of services required. If teachers are to perform at the level of competence demanded by society, they must continue to learn and grow professionally. Teachers, administrators, and parents must work together to determine major areas of need, and school systems must work with institutions of higher learning to provide appropriate growth opportunities. Specific incentives for training in high-priority areas need to be considered.

(Other personal factors and training deficits as discussed in Chapter V for administrators are also teacher stressors.)

SUMMARY

Teachers are currently looking closely at themselves and their profession. They are asking, "What am I teaching, how am I teaching, and why am I teaching?"

A conflict exists between the ideal and the real. Teachers are filled with idealistic hopes, but lack the skills and conditions necessary to achieve real goals. The motivation inspired by professional training or the need to meet the requirements of a new public law may only serve to frustrate teachers, who still must face the limitations of the classroom. Conflict between the desirable and the actual creates disillusionment and contributes to teacher burnout.

Instructor magazine ("Teacher Burnout," 1979b) devoted an entire issue to teacher burnout. Mortimer Feinberg, an industrial psychologist who has worked with many executives from the nation's largest corporations, was interviewed. When asked how he'd treat elementary teachers suffering from job burnout, Feinberg provided the following advice.*

> First we have to determine if the job depression is internalized. If you have trouble sleeping, no appetite or sexual drive, emotional outbursts of anger, you probably have internalized kinds of problems and need professional counseling. Maybe the solution is retirement or changing jobs. But if you're perfectly happy away from your job, then you know that it is an external problem and your job is getting to you. For these people we can do something. (p. 62)

Feinberg made the analogy of the mind and a tire. He said,

> If it isn't rotated it is going to wear out faster. To rotate the mind, don't have it constantly in the same gear. Maybe switch assignments for a year, Kindergarten this year, fourth grade next. But also, go beyond that, spend your leisure time with adults. Do something different evenings and summers.
>
>   It's important to build self esteem. Many industries have adopted the Japanese practice of a godfather—placing a person in charge of newer employees to inspire or teach, to act as a guardian. Schools could, and should adopt this practice. (p. 62)

Feinberg pointed out other ways to combat the effects of stress.

> Many industries spend a lot of money developing athletic facilities for its employees' after-hours use. Schools already have these facilities. A physical workout after school to limber tired muscles will go a great way toward eliminating mental weariness.
>
>   Finally, we—teachers, parents, the business community—must work toward raising the status of the teacher in the professional field. The public must perceive teachers as professionals as it did years ago. The health of our educational system depends on the effectiveness and

---

* Quoted with permission of Dr. Mortimer Feinberg.

mental attitudes of its teachers. We'll have fewer burned-out teachers when they begin to feel and assume their great influence and importance in the future of the nation. (p. 62)

Those who instruct our young deserve respect, support, and dignity. Teachers need to know that they are important and respected. Surveys have found that the majority of adults, when asked to identify the most significant person in their formative years, other than parents, usually named a teacher. The reality persists that the United States is still giving a better education to more children at all levels than any other country in the world.

CHAPTER VII

Prevention and
Remediation of Distress

Just as the maladaptive response to distress is a learned phenomenon, so can coping be learned or relearned. The mastery of distress is a process of managing future stress rather than responding inappropriately to a crisis (Burgoyne, 1975). Learning new responses is actually preventative rather than remedial, because it equips people to cope effectively on a long-term basis. However, learning to cope must be a personal process based upon how that particular individual perceives a stressor. Distress definitely fits the adage, "one man's poison is another man's cure." One school administrator may thrive on crisis, while another may become an insomniac in anticipation of a minor event. The major differences are related to personality, previous experiences, knowledge and awareness, degree of personal control, and the perceived importance of an event. For some, coping with stress (by avoiding distress) appears to be a gift or talent. For most, however, it can be a living hell.

LEARNING TO COPE WITH STRESS

Successful management of stress (coping) is primarily the process of converting the negative energy of an enemy into the positive energy of an ally—i.e., turning a potentially destructive stressor into a creative motivator. Stress is an enemy when it is excessive and becomes a handicap. Overstimulation or circuit-breaking distress can—as in a generator—be converted into adaptive energy through transfer or decompression. Like gasoline in an internal combustion engine, stress can be used in a controlled manner to provide optimum performance. With some training, most educators can get real mileage out of overstimulating or explosive job situations. If this destructive energy is harnessed, it can be mastered.

There are at least three primary factors (Adams, 1979) that mediate an individual's experience of distress: (1) the individual's personality, (2) his or her interpersonal environment, and (3) the nature of the organization in which he or she works. Adams and many other researchers strongly agree that changing one's distress-creating behaviors must be a gradual process. Wholesale life-style changes, like crash diets, are doomed to failure.

Obviously the first prerequisite to change is a strong commitment to change. The next step is establishment of a simple, manageable program for change. By slowly exchanging old habits for new ones, one can build a confident self-management program. It is very important that when a new stressor appears, one aggressively take the initiative toward positive and thoughtful change.

With any compulsive habit (drinking, overeating, smoking), a great deal of tension is reduced when a person is able to admit that he or she does in fact have a problem. Only after awareness and problem identification can one effectively establish a plan for coping. It is important to emphasize that the plan must be very personal and individualized. The secret of successful coping is not avoiding stress but learning to use adaptive energy wisely.

A key principle of distress management is a satisfying balance between work and play, challenge and leisure, distress and relaxation, struggling or taking it easy, companionship and solitude, discipline and self-indulgence. A life of balance and reasonable compromise requires understanding and planning. Understanding involves a positive attitude toward life's events and the ability to let provocation pass without undue reaction, but also without assuming a passive posture. Planning involves the maintenance of an optimal amount of stimulating stress, as well as prevention of stress overload. Most important is the realization that life provides choices, and the acceptance of responsibility for one's own behavior. This attitude is far more healthy than accepting the belief that life is predesigned and preprogrammed by outside forces.

Albrecht (1979) compared high-stress vs. low-stress life styles. An adaptation of his comparison appears in table 1:

TABLE 1
COMPARISON OF HIGH- AND LOW-STRESS LIFE STYLES

High-Stress Life Style	Low-Stress Life Style
1. Individual chronic unrelieved stress.	1. Individual accepts stress as a creative, challenging, and necessary phenomenon.
2. Is trapped into continuing stressful situations.	2. Has escape routes allowing for detachment and relaxation.
3. Struggles with people.	3. Asserts, negotiates, provides mutual respect, and establishes cooperative relations with people.
4. Engages in perceived distasteful, dull, unpleasant and unrewarding work.	4. Engages in challenging, satisfying, worthwhile work that offers intrinsic rewards.
5. Continually experiences time stress—too much to do in available time. (Time is the master.)	5. Maintains a well-balanced, challenging workload—periodic overload and crises are balanced by breathing periods. (Time is an ally.)
6. Worries about upcoming events.	6. Looks forward to positive events and balances threatening events with worthwhile goals.
7. Has poor health habits (lack of exercise, poor eating, drinking, smoking behavior).	7. Maintains some degree of physical fitness, eats well, and uses tobacco or alcohol sparingly.
8. Life activities are unbalanced (e.g., preoccupied with work or money or solitude).	8. Life activities are balanced by a variety of activities and interests that bring satisfaction.
9. Finds it difficult to relax or have a good time. Has unhealthy attitude about sex.	9. Finds pleasure in many daily activities and needs not "try hard to have a good time." Has healthy attitude about sex.
10. Sees life as serious and difficult. Has a weak sense of humor.	10. Enjoys life, can laugh at self, and has a good sense of humor.
11. Accepts high stress in a passive manner and suffers silently. Workaholic.	11. Re-engineers highly stressful situations beneficially and manages time effectively.

Note: Adapted from the book *Stress and the Manager* by Karl Albrecht. © 1979 by Prentice-Hall, Inc. Published by Prentice-Hall, Inc., Englewood Cliffs, N.J. 07632. Used by permission of the publisher.

The following techniques ("Self-Talk" and Social Support) represent the two most helpful methods of preventing and reducing distress.

DISPELLING FAULTY PERCEPTIONS THROUGH "SELF-TALK"

Stress, as discussed in Chapter I, is a perception. Distress is triggered by perceptions of threat to our well-being, and these perceptions can be based upon distorted or faulty beliefs. Distorted perceptions produce anger, frustration, and anxiety, because they structure the individual's view of the world. Typical examples of faulty perceptions or beliefs are:

1. Evaluating yourself as less worthy because you have fallen short of another's expectation.
2. Believing that others really don't care and that you're not very important.
3. Regarding yourself as inferior.
4. Feeling you are incapable of handling an extremely stressful situation.
5. Stereotyping others as bad because of isolated behaviors, or feeling you are the judge of how others must act.
6. Believing that worry is necessary in anticipating each future event.

Many philosophers and researchers feel that positive attitudes are the clearest way to self-respect, confidence, and successful inoculation against stress. For thousands of years writers have referred to thoughts as the cause agent of our actions:

Epictetus: "People are not upset by things but by their ideas about things."

Marcus Aurelius: "Our life is what our thoughts make it."

Shakespeare: "There is nothing either good or bad but thinking makes it so."

Milton: "The mind is its own place and in itself can make a heaven of hell, a hell of heaven."

Emerson: "The ancestor of every action is a thought—A man is what he thinks about all day long."

Thoreau: "Man is the artificer of his own happiness."

Lincoln: "Most folks are about as happy as they make up their minds to be."

Norman Vincent Peale: "You are not what you think you are; but what you *think*, you *are*."

In recent years, substantial research has been conducted to validate the importance of exercising personal control as a means of managing stress. Studies by Meichenbaum (1977) have shown that reactions to distress are in large part influenced by how a person cognitively appraises the stress. He has found significant differences between minimally distressed, as compared to highly distressed, individuals based on a single factor—their thinking styles and how they talk to themselves (self-talk).

Beck (1970) also found that those who suffered from severe stress were characterized by faulty beliefs expressed in self-verbalizations. He categorized the faulty beliefs into four areas: (1) dividing everything into opposites or extremes—"All of the other teachers are against me"; (2) making far-reaching generalizations—"My principal let me down. I'll never trust him again"; (3) viewing things in an exaggerated or magnified way, usually as catastrophic—"Why even try, it won't do any good, he's a waste"; (4) drawing conclusions without evidence, often in a self-recriminating way—"I goofed again, I'm just worthless."

The evidence strongly indicates that if a person feels even partially in control of a distressful situation, the negative effects of stress are reduced. If there is a feeling of no control or lack of predictability, people tend toward "learned helplessness." Fortunately, researchers like Albert Ellis (1973), in his development of Rational Emotive Therapy, have found that self-talk or inner dialogue can be turned to constructive use. He has developed methods for helping individuals to think differently and avoid negative feelings such as worry and fear (most often caused by mistaken or exaggerated beliefs). A person can extinguish old response patterns with the assistance of objective data, a sense of control, and revised self-talk. Maladaptive thinking patterns can be reversed by replacement with adaptive self-statements. Reversing failures, not rehearsing them, is one key to successful self-talk.

Confidence and trust in oneself comes first and foremost from inside, not from others. If one calls oneself incompetent or ineffective, he or she will act incompetently and ineffectively. If an individual believes him- or herself to be skilled and successful, others will share this confidence. Prevention of or coping with distress demands a positive attitude toward one's ability. Gaining an insight into mistaken beliefs is a starting point, because new beliefs evolve when old ones are proven incorrect.

The easiest method of determining one's own perceptions of situations is to write a summary of the stream of thoughts focused on a disturbing situation. One's self-talk will identify perceptions, beliefs, and fears. For example, when a deadline has to be met, does one use negative self-talk such as "I'll never get it done in time," "I'd better hurry or I'll never finish," or "I hate my job"? The underlying faulty belief may be, "I simply cannot handle deadlines. I'm never prepared and never have enough time."

If this is the case, one can take the following, positive self-talk approach. Replace the negative thought pattern with another one such as, "I'll just take one thing at a time until I get it done. Some pressures are anticipated on this job, and this is one of them. I really am capable of completing this on time." Remember, many of the thoughts one has have become so automatic that unless they are examined carefully one can fall prey to false beliefs established years ago.

The construct in table 2 provides comparative examples of positive and negative self-talk, and the results of each type of interior monologue.

TABLE 2

EXAMPLES OF SELF-TALK
ILLUSTRATED BY MR. DISTRESSED AND MR. CALM

Potential Stressors	Mr. Distressed (Stressed, Ineffective Response)	Mr. Calm (Relaxed, Effective Response)
1. 7:00 A.M. Alarm did not go off. Overslept.	"I've got to hurry. I don't have time for a shower or breakfast. I can't be late. I'll never get things done."	"This is not a big problem. If I take my time I may be a few minutes late, but I'll make it up. I'll just have something light to eat. I want to be fresh when I get to work"
	Results Left home in a hurried, anxious state.	*Results* Left home in a calm state.
2. 7:55 A.M. Traffic jam.	"These ♯ ✳ ? ⌇ drivers. I don't know where they learned to drive. Don't they know I'm late? Why can't he get in the slow lane—idiot."	"I'll just let the traffic end and proceed normally. There's nothing to worry about. Things are under control. Why worry? I can't do a thing about it."
	Results Blood pressure and pulse rate rose. Arrived at work hurried and harried.	*Results* Remained calm and relaxed. Arrived at work fresh and alert.

(Continued on next page)

Table 2 (continued)

Potential Stressors	Mr. Distressed (Stressed, Ineffective Response)	Mr. Calm (Relaxed, Effective Response)
3. 11:00 A.M. Unappreciative boss.	"This isn't what I need today. My boss knows that I put in 100 hours on that project. I should get credit." *Results* Stormed out of the office angry and frustrated.	"Beneath all this hostility the boss does have a point. I can take care of this problem now before it gets more serious. I will talk to the boss and explain the personal involvement I've had in it and how important it is to me." *Results* Problem resolved after mutual concerns were expressed.
4. 12:00 Noon Behind Schedule	"I don't know if I'll ever get through this paper work. I'll forget lunch and get it all done." *Results* Made mistakes in work because of frenetic, unrelenting pace.	"I think I'll visit the antique store down the road and then take my bag lunch to the park. It will refresh me." *Results* Came back after lunch in a refreshed mood and was better able to concentrate.
5. 10:30 P.M. Bedtime.	"There are so many things going through my mind I can't sleep. Maybe I'll try counting sheep." *Results* Awoke exhausted, unhappy, and frustrated.	"I'll go to bed a little early tonight and get a good night's sleep. I accomplished a lot today. *Results* Awoke early, renewed and pleasant.

Rules of Negative Self-talk (Self-talk Killers)

- Become convinced that the only alternative to your problem behavior is to go to the other extreme.
- Assume others do not listen and that nothing you could say or do will change the situation.
- Assume that others will get angry, and will think you are crazy, foolish, or too critical.

- Believe that others can read your mind or recognize your subtle hints, so that you don't have to tell them what you are feeling.
- Feel that trying once is enough.
- Believe that making a mistake proves you are less of a person; convince yourself that you must be perfect in all that you try to do.

SOCIAL SUPPORT

Social support has been identified as the single most effective means of preventing or ameliorating the effects of occupational stress. Research literature is replete with citations identifying social support as the number one antidote for distress.

Social support is defined as a relationship with one or more people characterized by frequent interactions of a strongly positive nature—especially interactions that lend emotional assistance. It is symbolized by trust, empathy, and mutual concern. Social support has been studied as a major distress antidote for less than a decade. Although empirical data is limited, that which exists strongly suggests that supportive social relationships with superiors, colleagues, and subordinates at work directly reduce levels of occupational stress. Support satisfies important personal and social needs and makes workers feel more positive about themselves. Social support also reduces role conflict and ambiguity. Cassel (1976) has suggested an analogy between the buffering effect of support and other processes such as immunization and proper nutrition, which increase one's resistance to disease.

It is necessary that one recognize his or her own need for human closeness and mutual strength. Social support provides an opportunity to express feelings, obtain advice and guidance, give and receive assistance in problem solving, laugh, cry, and share. Not only does it provide catharsis, but in the process it allows for constructive feedback from others.

Organizations can assist by supporting either informal or formal programs among employees. Distress rates are lower for individuals who actively express their feelings to colleagues. Surprisingly, what individuals may have felt to be their singular concern is shared by others. Mutual expression of feelings and ideas about similar concerns can serve as a yardstick for comparison. Sharing also provides valuable information on others' reactions to stressful situations. Most importantly, it provides positive feedback often lacking within the organizational structure.

Considerable research evidence indicates that the support of other people eases one's perception of negative situations. Social support can buffer the effect of potential distress by helping the person to perceive a stressor as less threatening. Researchers have found that anxiety over work-related matters decreases as cohesiveness within the work group increases (Seashore, 1954; Likert, 1961; Kahn et al., 1964). In a study of heart disease risk factors among administrators (Caplan, 1971), it was found that those who report poor relations with their subordinates (low social support) are also subject to work overload and role ambiguity, possess significant amounts of serum cholesterol and serum glucose, suffer from high blood pressure, and are addicted to smoking. Among those having good relations with others (high social support), there are no significant cardiovascular or related risk factors.

Maslach (1976), Freudenberger (1976), and Mattingly (1977) all have expressed the strong belief that support from colleagues and an opportunity to express feelings at the work place significantly help the worker to cope with stress. Willingness, confidentiality, and honesty with peers without collusion are all required factors. All who work together for the same social purpose must assist each other in every way possible.

House and Wells (1977) found that the social support derived from a "significant other" can be quite effective in mitigating the effects of distress on health. They expressed a strong belief that work supervisors provide an especially appealing focus for the provision of social support. Not only are supervisors capable, but they also have organizational influence. Spouses can also be an important source of support. In some work situations social support may not only contribute to the direct reduction of occupational stress, but also provides resistance and an immunizing effect for employees. Social support is best provided by multiple sources. A work support system can provide job-related awareness and technical help. "Like colleagues" within the school environment experience the same daily, distressful conditions. They can share these experiences directly, as well as provide new ideas, suggestions, or on-the-spot advice necessary for more successful coping.

At home, a spouse can lend a welcome ear and offer emotional support. Friends in similar occupations can also provide support by acting as a sounding board. Having two or more support systems provides for more objective sources of strength. Unfortunately, Don Quixote is not the only one whose effectiveness was handicapped by ignoring this rule.

Although social support cannot be considered a substitute for the reduction of occupational stress, it can be used as a means of alleviating the effect of such stress. LaRocco and Jones (1978) recommended the direct removal of occupational stress as the major means of stress control.

A note of caution is in order, however. Any group—formal or informal—which is established to provide mutual social support should formulate a set of rules based upon the research findings for group dynamics. For example, the optimum number is three to eight participants. The rules might also place limits on unproductive responses, by setting a time limit on "griping."

METHODS OF RELAXATION TRAINING

The Greek philosopher Plato recommended in the *Republic* that the body, mind, and spirit be viewed as a single unit rather than as separate entities. Plato felt that education of the mind and body together produced harmonious development of the human character and spirit. There are many mind-body-spirit activities that have individually proven valuable in preventing stress from becoming distressful. The following pages include a number of preventative and remedial activities.

Physical Activity

Job stress is no longer considered to be a problem related only to jobs such as those done by air traffic controllers or executives. It is now recognized that all jobs produce various levels of stress.

Cofer and Appley (1964) reported that all human beings act irrationally or unreasonably at times. As stress arousal increases, deteriorative effects become noticeable in a number of performance areas. There is a tendency toward rigidity, inflexibility, inability to profit from experience, suspiciousness, hostility, irritability, increased errors, and decreased performance.

According to Greenberg (1980) a number of behaviors may occur. They include: not seeing other alternatives; making less sensible decisions, not considering ultimate consequences; narrowed points of view (tunnel vision); poorer quality and less productive output; wasting time and activity; lack of creativity, irrational actions, poorer listening; making unnecessary mistakes.

In addition to decreased work productivity, the body also undergoes physiological change. The autonomic nervous system reacts to distress by accelerating the heart beat, increasing blood pressure and sugar level (from the liver), diverting blood from the skin to the heart and brain, increasing respiration, emergency hormones and muscle tension. The purpose of these changes is to prepare the individual for fight or flight.

Both responses demand physical activity—reactions which date back almost one million years of human evolution. This relatively primitive nervous system becomes short circuited when muscle activity does not burn up the additional fuel (sugar) and cholesterol, while reducing respiration, heart rate, hormone levels and blood pressure. Consequently a balanced state is not achieved and physiological damage is likely to occur in one or more organs or systems.

These facts are rarely realized when we are irrational, unreasonable, or mistake prone. Intellectual impairment, performance decrements, and lack of normal physiological responses create a cycle that escalates distress and produces harmful effects on body parts.

Since the body automatically prepares itself for action in a stress-provoking situation, it is advisable for the individual involved to engage in some type of activity to provide necessary balance. The relief provided by physical activity is amazingly effective. Almost always following a brisk walk, game of tennis, isometrics, gardening, etc., the response is positive and successful. Examples: "I feel so much better," or "I'm much more calm." "I'm no longer upset."

Meditation

There are literally hundreds of methods of meditation, which is perhaps the oldest of all mind-body techniques. Eastern religions have used meditation for thousands of years. Western religions similarly use meditation in the form of prayer. Each technique basically produces deep muscle and mental relaxation. Recently the most popular form has been transcendental meditation (TM). This is a passive mental process of focusing on a "mantra" (single word or number) for approximately 15 to 20 minutes. For tense people, it has been found that it's best to start with progressive muscle relaxation and then move into TM. It is suggested that if the mind wanders it should be brought back to the mantra.

Frew (1977) concluded that reduction of stress through TM is associated with increased productivity and efficiency at work. He wrote, "People who operate at relatively low levels of stress appear to enjoy their work, to get along better with other people and to be more effective at their jobs" (p. 175). According to McGaffey (1978), over 120 U.S. companies have provided their employees an opportunity to learn transcendental meditation. Some companies even provide special rooms for meditation.

In his book *The Relaxation Response* (1975), Dr. Herbert Benson of Harvard has popularized the use of transcendental meditation. He has conducted extensive research and shown the benefits (particularly the lowering of blood pressure) of TM. Benson has demonstrated that just as the body has a fight-or-flight response (sympathetic nervous system), it also has an innate compensatory relaxation response (parasympathetic nervous system) which can be produced by meditation.

Dr. Benson has suggested in the *Harvard Business Review* that organizations should provide an alternative to the coffee break—the TM relaxation break. A deluge of protest letters called him outrageous and said stress was necessary for business management. Since then companies like AT&T and General Foods have found tremendous value in such an approach. Instead of using a mantra, he uses a non-cult technique which he calls a "mental device." His suggested mental device is to repeat the word "one."

Benson's method is as follows: find a comfortable position in a quiet environment, close your eyes, assume a passive attitude (the most difficult element), while concentrating on a word deeply relax all of your muscles, breathe through your nose repeating the word. This form of meditation requires about 40 minutes a day—20 minutes in the morning and 20 minutes in the late afternoon. Dr. Benson stresses adopting a passive attitude rather than trying to bring about the desired physiological reaction. Transcendental meditation involves the following procedures:

- Choose a quiet environment with few distractions. Sit in a comfortable position so there is no undue muscle tension. Avoid lying down; there is a tendency to fall asleep.
- Close your eyes.
- Deeply relax all your muscles, beginning at your feet and progressing up to your face. Keep them relaxed.
- Breathe through your nose. Become aware of your breathing. As you breathe out, say the word, "ONE," silently to yourself. For example, breathe in . . . out, "ONE"; in . . . out, "ONE," etc. Breathe easily and naturally. The repetition of "ONE" helps break the train of distracting thoughts; attention to the normal rhythm of breathing enhances the repetition.
- Continue for 10 to 20 minutes. You may open your eyes to check

the time, but do not use an alarm. When you finish, sit quietly for
several minutes, at first with your eyes closed and later with your
eyes opened.

- Do not worry about whether you are successful in achieving a deep
  level of relaxation. Adopt a passive, "let-it-happen" attitude and
  permit relaxation to occur at its own pace. When distracting
  thoughts occur, try to ignore them and return to repeating "ONE."
  With practice, the response should come with little effort. Practice
  the technique once or twice daily, but not within two hours after
  any meal, since the digestive process seems to interfere with it.

Progressive Relaxation

Progressive relaxation was developed by Dr. Edmund Jacobson to
combat the effects of stress. This approach requires the participant to
first tense and then relax muscles in the body, with special emphasis
on the recognition of tenseness and the ability to relax at the onset
of stress. The method is termed "progressive" because it starts with
muscles in one part of the body and proceeds to all other parts. Begin
by relaxing the muscles of your right foot, then the left foot, and proceed upwards, tensing and relaxing every muscle group up to the top
of your head.

Thought-Intrusion Exercises

Intrusive thoughts racing through one's head can be a persistent
interference with relaxation. Several methods of achieving a relaxed
state are available:

- Efforts to fight off intrusive ideas are often ineffective. Let them flow
  without resistance. At the same time, focus on a pleasant, calm, past
  experience, a word or number, or count backwards from 50.
- If the above process is ineffective and thoughts persist after several
  passive attempts to dissolve them, say "No!" Use this self-command
  repeatedly over a five- to ten-minute period while remaining in a
  state of deep muscle and mental relaxation.
- A third approach is to imagine a pleasant scene such as a mountain
  lake, a calm ocean, or a blue sky with white drifting clouds. Focus
  on the scene to replace the intrusive thoughts. As this proceeds, let
  the pleasant scene fade and let a gray or black nothingness perme-
  ate your closed eyes. Ignore any other visual detail. Finally, let the
  blue colors (lake, sky, ocean) drift back in. Hold on to the calmness
  that the blue colors represent. Savor this state of mental relaxation.

Focusing on Breathing

Given practice, these simple exercises have a potent effect as circuit breakers for distress.

A short relaxation exercise:

- Close your eyes.
- Count backwards from ten.
- Inhale on each count, saying to yourself, "I am . . ."
- Exhale on each count, saying, "calm and relaxed."

A longer relaxation exercise:

- Sit, lie, or stand comfortably.
- Imagine a pleasant, quiet place that represents your ideal location for physical and mental relaxation.
- Draw a deep breath and hold it for five seconds, exhale slowly, and tell your muscles to relax. Let your jaw, tongue, and mouth drop with the feeling of relaxation.
- Feel the energy go up and down like a bicycle chain as you inhale and exhale. Think about the long, deep breaths into your stomach and feel the calmness and peacefulness. Imagine your whole body and mind being renewed and refreshed.
- Think of inhaling invigorating, pure, new air and exhaling old, less clean air.
- After one to three minutes, slowly open your eyes and stretch. You may return to your place of relaxation whenever you desire to experience peace and calm.

Other relaxation exercises:

Count backwards from 50. You can get yourself into an almost totally relaxed state within five minutes. In this stage give yourself a personal message such as, "I will be more calm," or, "I am relaxed and at peace in my world."

When an opportunity becomes available, breathe with the stomach (feel it move in and out) for a few slow breaths. Practice it at odd moments during the day. By taking three or four deep breaths and focusing all of your attention into the relaxation of breathing, relief will be only a few seconds away.

Stretch your arms toward the sky. Take a deep breath and extend your arms and torso as high as you can. Count to five. Exhale with an audible sigh of relief. Do this three to five times.

With your middle and forefinger or thumb find the pulse on your wrist or lower neck. Regulate your breathing with your pulse rate. Breathe out every six pulses. Continue for about three minutes.

Gently place your thumb over one nostril. Slowly draw ten deep breaths. Switch nostrils and repeat ten more breaths. Now slowly inhale through both nostrils. Exhale through your mouth. Focus on your breathing. Place your palm on your diaphragm; feel it expand as you inhale slowly and deeply. Feel it contract as you slowly exhale. Express a quiet but audible sigh of relief with each breath. Continue for three to five minutes.

Gently hold your thumbs or forefingers over your ears. Close your eyes and listen to the sounds of your body. Listen for the harmony of your inner sounds, particularly the rhythm of your breathing.

Densensitization

The process of desensitization was developed by behavioral psychologists as a technique to reprogram one's reactions in fearful or troublesome situations. The fear of heights, giving a speech, taking a test, enclosed areas, animals (dogs, spiders, rats), or an impending crisis are common and real stressors. Desensitization is basically the use of relaxing conditions combined with rehearsal of progressively more difficult situations.

By beginning in a relaxed state, one carefully rehearses the aversive situation, each time gradually reducing the anxiety. Visualization of the situation begins with simple steps. For example, giving a speech might first involve going to the library to collect information, next organizing the information, and then writing the speech. Rehearsing in preparation for the speech might be next: first rehearse in front of someone with whom you are close; later rehearse with one or two people in mind whom you know slightly less well; finally, rehearse mentally before the actual group to which you are to speak.

Desensitization, like any relaxation process, works better when it is practiced often. If giving a speech in class is traumatic, it may take lots of trials under gradually more formal conditions. If at any point in the process one becomes even slightly stressed, he or she should stop immediately and backtrack to the previous step. Positive feedback (from self and others) is necessary and important throughout each step. If the fear or anxiety is highly entrenched, professional assistance may be necessary.

Desensitization is programmed relearning that has shown remarkably positive results in both clinical and laboratory settings.

Mental Relaxation

- First, relax your muscles.
- You are now ready to begin a mind-clearing process that deepens relaxation.
- Enter a passive state—let your thoughts flow freely.
- Become aware of your slow, deep breathing. Follow each deep breath closely.
- If thoughts still come to mind, think them, and then slowly put full attention back on your breathing.
- Feel the clear, brisk air fill your lungs and feel waves of relaxation as you expel each breath.
- Imagine a blue sky, the sea, or a calm object.
- If you still do not feel calm and restful, it is helpful to repeat a soothing word (love, peace) or a neutral word (one, there, now). If a word distracts you, use a meaningless sound or syllable (e.g., yi, tr).
- Remind yourself to keep the muscles of your neck, face, eyes, and forehead relaxed.

Yoga Exercise

The Yoga Shavasan Exercise was developed by K. K. Datey (Lamott, 1974) as an exercise to let go and relax. It is a relatively easy exercise and frequently found to be pleasant.

Take off your necktie, shoes, and any other constricting clothing. Lie on your back with your legs sprawling apart and your arms lying easily beside you but not touching your body. Datey says that your legs should be spread at an angle of 30 degrees and your arms at 15 degrees.

Close your eyes, not squeezing them shut, but letting your eyelids droop. Let your fingers lie in a natural, half-curled position. Breathe regularly, breathing with your stomach rather than with your chest. Learn to breathe rhythmically in such a way that each inhalation is followed by a pause and each exhalation by a longer pause. This can be achieved by breathing to a slow count of seven, like this:

> One, two—inhale
> Three—hold
> Four, five—exhale
> Six, seven—hold
> One, two—inhale again.

You should soon fall into such a regular rhythm of breathing that you hardly need to count. Counting, however, will keep your mind aware of what is going on in your body and will protect you from the intrusion of disturbing thoughts from the outside world. If you find you are breathing through your nostrils regularly without counting, think of the coolness of air as it enters your nostrils and the warmth of the air as it leaves. Imagine that your arms and legs are becoming heavier and heavier and warmer and warmer. Then go back to the seven counts. Datey recommends Shavasan for 30 minutes a day.

Biofeedback

Biofeedback is a technique using equipment that measures mind-body functions (muscle tension, intestinal activity, blood flow, breathing, heartbeat). This monitoring program tells us what is going on in our body with regard to a particular function. Our five senses are used as monitors. For example, if we take the function of muscle tension, with the aid of equipment we could hear the activity of increased or decreased tension, as well as see the machine register minute changes (millionths of a volt) in our muscle activity. With heartbeat, we can hear how fast it is or see whether it changes rate. After general awareness, one is taught how to change these functions with the assistance of instantaneous feedback of biological data.

Biofeedback is simply an electronically assisted means of awareness and change of bodily functions within our control. It is no different from a baby learning how to put food in its mouth. Using the feedback of results and continued practice, the baby eventually learns how to hit the mouth on the first try. A mirror is another form of feedback. By looking into a mirror we receive feedback about our smile, frown, or the neatness of our hair. This tells us whether an adjustment is needed or not. With practice we may need a mirror less and less.

If we choose a bodily function that may be dysfunctional due to distress, we proceed to monitor it by amplifying the bodily function and making it accessible to our sense organs. We can now tell what is going on immediately and continuously. Then we go about changing this dysfunctional behavior by learning new and more appropriate adaptive behaviors. Any bodily function that can be monitored can be changed.

It is not unusual for people to make significant changes in their physiologically adaptive mechanisms. Changes in breathing, heartbeat, muscle tension, acidity, and blood pressure are often dramatic, and with practice can become long term. Three-fourths of all medical complaints are related to distress (Shealley, 1977). This does not mean that there is anything permanently wrong with the body, but the symptoms indicate that the body is temporarily out of balance. Muscles may be tight, blood pressure high, or stomach acid levels elevated. All of these may be learned dysfunctions capable of being prevented or remediated. Change occurs through awareness, monitoring, and relearning of unhealthy responses.

Although used in major hospitals (UCLA, Columbia, Menninger, Mayo, and many others) biofeedback is still in its initial stages of development. Some companies such as TRW have used individual and group biofeedback techniques, with excellent results, for such ailments as migraine headaches.

Biofeedback basically teaches people to recognize their own physiology and changes in their bodies. If one is aware of body conditions, something can be done about them. It is a natural means of learning that assists in recognizing clues and signals that go on within us. Learning to relieve these symptoms helps us to be healthier.

One executive (West, 1978) suggested that "maybe in the future corporations will require their top executives to undergo biofeedback training just as you expect them to pursue educational or professional studies" (p. 7).

Deep Muscle Relaxation

Deep relaxation is a profoundly restful condition. People who reach this state generally report feelings of peacefulness, optimism, kindliness, inspiration, and cheerfulness. Psychologists also note profound changes in breathing, heart rate, blood pressure, and blood chemistry following the deep relaxation exercises described below:

- Take a 15-minute break.
- Find a quiet environment and lie on your back or sit comfortably; close your eyes and become passive.
- For right-handed people, begin by physically tensing the right hand for an instant, then relax and let it go limp. Tell it to be heavy and warm. Continue with the rest of the right side of the body, moving up to the forearm, upper arm, shoulder, then down to the foot, lower leg, and upper leg. Next, follow the same procedure on the left side of the body. (If you are left-handed, begin the procedure with the left hand and continue.) The hands, arms, and legs are

now relaxed, heavy, and warm. Wait for these feelings to arise. (After mastering the technique, you will not need to tense the muscles before relaxing them.)

- Next, relax the muscles of the hips and let a wave of relaxation pass up from the abdomen to the chest. Do not tense these muscles. Tell them to be heavy and warm. Your breathing will come more from the diaphragm and will be slower. Wait for this breathing change.
- Now let the wave of relaxation continue into the shoulders, neck, jaw, and muscles of the face. Pay special attention to the muscles controlling the eyes and forehead. Let your jaw hang open.
- Practice this drill twice daily: 15 to 20 minutes is ideal (but even three minutes is better than nothing when circumstances do not permit a longer session). Practice before meals or no sooner than one hour after meals. You can also practice before an anticipated stress experience, but no more frequently than four times a day.
- If you are not sure whether or not you are relaxed, ask another person to raise your arm or leg about five inches and then let go. If it drops like a dead weight, you are relaxed.
- With practice you will learn to attain deep muscle relaxation—the feeling of heavy, warm, inert muscles—in as short a time as two minutes.
- Many people are surprised how deep a state of relaxation they find with continued practice.
- Keep a log of your responses after you have practiced deep relaxation.

Various relaxation tapes are also available. What has proven most helpful, however, is to tape the sequence above or other exercises in your own voice.

Autogenic Training

Originating in the 1890s in Germany, autogenic training was developed by Johannes Schultz. Autogenic training is based on autohypnotic methods; it induces body changes—such as a heavy feeling, warmth, regular heartbeat, and slow, regular breathing—that occur when we are very quiet. Studies (Luthe, 1970) have indicated that autogenic training does decrease heart rate, blood pressure, and respiratory rate. Thus it does influence and assist the functions of the body to achieve a state of equilibrium. It basically involves concentration on mental images, relaxation, and self-talk. The exercises are listed below:

- Sit quietly with eyes closed at the edge of a chair (loosen clothing and remove watch and eyeglasses for comfort).
- Sense the state of your muscles.
- Let yourself collapse in the chair like a rag doll (i.e., back rounded, head forward, hands comfortable on knees).
- Concentrate on your dominant arm and allow it to become very heavy. Do the same with your other arm, focusing on the heaviness and intensifying it as much as possible.
- Relax your legs in a similar way.
- Return to your dominant arm and feel the heat grow until it is very warm and pleasant. Continue with your other arm and then each leg.
- Keep close and continuous concentration on your arms, legs, and body. Feel the heaviness and warmth as they increase and spread.

One can measure the effectiveness of this technique using a simple thermometer. By placing the thermometer gently against your dominant middle finger prior to the exercise and again afterwards, the effects of autogenic training can be determined. After practice your finger temperature should have risen, indicating that the smooth muscles have relaxed the capillaries at the surface of your hand. This allows the capillaries to carry more blood, and thus reduces blood pressure and increases circulation.

Tape-recording your own voice to the Schultz "self-talk" formula is helpful in creating your own autogenic training. Using a soft, slow, deliberate manner, speak into the microphone leaving long pauses between the following phrases.

I feel quite quiet.
I am beginning to feel quite relaxed.
My feet feel heavy and relaxed.
My ankles, my knees, and my hips feel heavy, relaxed, and comfortable.
My solar plexus and the whole central portion of my body feel relaxed and quiet.
My hands, my arms, and my shoulders feel heavy, relaxed, and comfortable.
My neck, my jaws, and my forehead feel relaxed.
They feel comfortable and smooth.
My whole body feels quiet, heavy, comfortable, and relaxed.
I feel quite relaxed.
My arms and hands are heavy and warm.
I feel quite quiet.

> My whole body is relaxed and my hands are warm . . . relaxed and
> warm.
> Warmth is flowing into my hands, they are warm . . . warm.

Listen to each phrase and then repeat it to yourself silently. As you say, "My feet feel heavy and relaxed," imagine that your feet are turning into sacks of cement. As you say, "My arms and hands are heavy and warm," imagine your hands lying in a pan of soapy, steaming water. When the tape is through, take your finger temperature again.

Don't be surprised or distressed if at first your temperature shows no change or actually goes down. Don't try to force the results. Play the tape every day—better yet, play it morning and evening—remembering to take your finger temperature before and after. In a few days you will find that the temperature is rising—two degrees, four degrees, six degrees, and eventually as much as ten degrees. As your hands warm up, your sense of body tension will diminish.

SUMMARY

Just as tension is a learned response to distress, so can relaxation become a learned preventative approach. The mastery of distress involves managing future stress (before it becomes distress), rather than letting it build up to the point of crisis. Although individual differences exist, everyone can develop appropriate coping skills. Coping begins with awareness of symptoms and causes and a commitment to change. Establishing goals and simple, manageable objectives can result in slowly exchanging old unsuccessful habits for new energy-conserving ones. A happy compromise between tension and ease, work and play, can be obtained by harnessing the stimulating force of stress. Control over one's mind, body, and external environment is the only known path to successful renewal. An individual can take major responsibility for his or her behavior by using appropriate self-talk (mind), developing multiple social support systems (environment), and relaxing prior to or at the onset of unnecessary muscle tension (body).

CHAPTER VIII

An Individualized
Stress Management Program

BASIC ELEMENTS AND
TECHNIQUES OF STRESS MANAGEMENT

It is extremely difficult for a person without skills or information to manage distress. There are many ways to prevent or ameliorate its negative effects, however, given the proper tools. Almost all management programs begin with awareness and self-assessment. A harried school principal or distressed teacher can begin a successful revitalization by first recognizing and identifying the troubled situation. Awareness alone can sometimes lead to self-change. If, in fact, distress is a perceived inability to cope, awareness of new coping strategies can in itself allay some of the feeling of helplessness. As awareness grows, the individual can learn to practice coping techniques at the first sign of impending distress.

By paying close attention to both mind and body, and by becoming familiar with the signals aroused within, a person can begin a distress management program. If one is continually aware of bodily changes, he or she will be better able to make immediate adjustments. If a person feels shoulder and neck muscles becoming tense, experiences low back pain, gets a headache, has a need for antacid medication, or feels confused and unable to focus his or her attention, it is important to determine the event(s) that caused the distress reaction. Once symptoms are identified, causes can likewise be clarified and new responses can be made in order to short-circuit distress.

The development of an individualized distress management plan involves stress awareness, problem identification, commitment to change, goal setting, self-observation, relaxation, self-talk, imagery, and repeated practice. The plan must also be tailored to fulfill individual needs. Set initial goals in the form of small incremental steps. Don't fall victim to a half-hearted effort; stick to the plan for at least six weeks. Don't let up and don't vary the pattern until habituation occurs. The skills that are developed will act as a genuine antidote to the effects of distress.

It is important to remember that skills are learned and must be practiced. Think of distress management as analogous to physical exercise. If one wishes to become physically fit, one must continue a fitness program faithfully. More battles are lost from lack of persistence than any other factor. Each person should talk to him- or herself in the following way: "I am strong, I am capable, and I will succeed— I can do it."

A useful self-management technique is to identify environmental distressors. For example, clock watching (or frequent glances at a wristwatch), telephone calls, or a certain pile on an office desk may become in themselves distress enhancers. A relatively simple technique is to use gummed stars, decals, or colored pencil marks to identify these items. Each time one looks at the clock or telephone, it will serve as a reminder to pause a few seconds, take a deep breath and relax, or to use a relaxation technique (described in Chapter VII). It is important to change to somewhat different cues about every six weeks, because of a tendency to satiate and then ignore the cues. Also, it is often helpful to have an enlarged photo or a poster to look at or some calming music to listen to when bodily reminders signal the beginning of distress.

A study of successful executives (Berry, 1977) pointed out several key characteristics of effective, individualized distress management. Berry found that success begins with self-analysis of one's current position and needs. The next step involves establishing short- and long-term goals and preparing a self-development program that includes follow-up and needed "course corrections" as one proceeds.

The basic elements of a distress management program include:

- Identify the kinds of stress one experiences. Ask oneself, "What two major stressors are affecting me most? Under what conditions or within what specific environment do I feel the most distress? What do I say to myself when I am under extreme pressure?"
- For six weeks keep a daily log of stressful events. Record what occurred prior to those feelings, the time of day, the actual feeling

and the responses to each stressful situation. Spend time differentiating perceptions of real threats from faulty beliefs. Then, rate each day on a scale of one (disaster) to ten (a cinch). Individuals using this approach usually find that the good days quickly begin to outnumber the bad.

- Rudyard Kipling said, "I keep six honest serving men. They taught me all I know. Their names are what and why and when and how and where and who." It is extremely important to collect the facts, analyze them, and then develop a plan of action. Benjamin Franklin used this technique to discover 13 personal faults (e.g., wasting time, arguing or contradicting others, and being concerned over trivia). He realized he needed to correct these faults, so each night he gave himself a severe "going over." He set out to correct them one at a time. Once a fault was mastered, he moved on to the next. His battle lasted some two years.
- If distress is perceived by a number of persons in the organization, get an expert to identify the specific causes of distress. Analyze the distribution of authority and responsibility in the organization. Evaluate work load and levels of communication or feedback. Companies such as Dupont, Dow, and others use consulting firms such as Cardiometrics and Executive Health Examiners to assist with stress problems. They have frequently found middle management to be a hotbed of occupational stress (Gibson, 1977).

The outside experts' approach should be dedicated to the detection, identification, education, referral, treatment, and follow up of troubled organizations or employees (Mancuso, 1979). Other companies such as IBM, Ford, Xerox, and Honeywell are initiating internal programs to help managers cope with stress ("How Companies Cope with Executive Stress," 1978). These programs begin by making executives aware of what causes distress and how to cope more effectively. Meditation, biofeedback (preferred by executives), and progressive relaxation are major ingredients in these programs.

- Be able to read your own symptoms of distress. Such signals might include: defensiveness, excessive paper work, extremely active or lethargic behavior, withdrawal and aloofness, or irrational behavior (anger, refusal, extreme resistance to change, complaints). Be particularly aware of communicative responses. For example, a person monopolizing a conversation may be trying too hard and not paying attention to ideas, needs, and possible solutions from others.
- Once identified, distress can be handled by means of an individual distress-management program using any number of coping tech-

niques described in this chapter. A simple, ten-second relaxation exercise, deep breathing, a sensible distraction or short "time out" often help prevent distress reactions. If one anticipates a particularly stressful day, it may help to wear favorite clothes, take time for a relaxation break, or ask for a supportive, friendly ear. Rewarding oneself with a pleasurable experience (e.g., dinner with spouse or close friend) after a tough day makes it more worthwhile.

- Know when to pull back and relax to avoid fights or unnecessary flight. Withdrawal or anger only fuels distress. Be aware that people become prone to health problems once they exceed their capacity to cope with stress. Try to forget everything that is ugly or painful.
- Recognize the fact that no person will be liked or loved by everyone. Remember the adage "Don't waste time befriending a mad dog." Likewise, don't attempt to change an impossible situation, because frustration will paralyze one's efficiency and instead create more distress.

As part of a three-year longitudinal study of management stress, Howard, Rechnitzer, and Cunningham (1975) identified the five most effective techniques for coping with job tension. They are:

1. Build resistance by regular sleep and good health habits.
2. Compartmentalize work and nonwork life.
3. Engage in physical exercise.
4. Talk through the situation with peers on the job.
5. Withdraw temporarily from the situation.

They also found that low-stress group members (those most successful in coping with distress) have an action-oriented, preventative concern about distress, a greater awareness of their psycho-physiological capacities, and a problem-solving orientation to issues causing job tensions. This low-stress group seems to know the kind of job situations that produce distress; they also know when they are under stress and what to do about it. On the other hand, the high-stress group simply worked harder under stress by (metaphorically speaking) pushing down further on the accelerator.

In the following pages many individual prescriptions are presented. Although various possible solutions are offered, it is not the intent of the author to suggest that every one be used. First of all, each individual is different. A method that works for one person may not work for another. Every individual will need his or her own custom-fitted approach. Second and equally important, no one should attempt a distress management program that adds more stress. Trying to accomplish too much too quickly not only results in failure, but also adds a substantial amount of new stress. To eliminate frustration and overload, only a few prescriptive solutions should be attempted at a time. It is suggested that after these new approaches have become habitual (usually within six weeks), then other approaches can be introduced. Remember, real long-term growth is gradual. Overnight changes—like most New Year's resolutions—almost never succeed.

PERSONAL PRESCRIPTIONS
FOR GAINING CONTROL OVER ONE'S DESTINY

Conquering Time Sickness

Type A personalities* have never learned to accommodate to the stress of time. This personality constellation is often described as a human time bomb. Learning to live by the day and not by the minute is a first step in eliminating time sickness. Too many people put overemphasis on their minute-to-minute activities. Sound planning involves much longer spans of time. Acceptance of this simple concept helps individuals to consider time as relative to a lifetime and not to a particular hour of the day. Minutes tick away meaninglessly if one focuses on a wristwatch and forgets the totality of life.

In overcoming time sickness, it is helpful to regularize one's environment. The same stressors will be more manageable and therefore less harmful if they occur predictably. One should arrange an individual schedule to accommodate situations of high stress, providing more control over the events of life. One should strive to become the master of time rather than its slave.

Life is like an hourglass: we can't force more than one grain of sand through its narrow neck at a time without breaking it. Each day we have a myriad of tasks to accomplish, but if we don't take them one at a time, we are bound to exceed our physical or mental limits. Remember, half the hospital beds in the United States are filled with people who collapsed under excessive stress. Take one day and one task at a time.

Leaving time between activities and scheduling only as many tasks as can reasonably be completed without feeling overwhelmed are necessary for personal survival. Learning to slow down—especially while walking, talking, and eating—and finding time each day to re-

---

* For a description of Type A personalities, see Chapter II and Appendix B.

lax, exercise, meditate, and quietly think are important keys to successful living.

Time Management

Without proper time management, work can become a rapid succession of deadlines. Lakein (1973), a major pioneer of time management techniques, developed a system for setting priorities and using time as an ally rather than as one's master. He asserted that the major task of time management is to develop a ranked list of things "to do." The "to do" list provides an opportunity to add or delete items based upon one's perception of priority (high, medium, or low). Crossing off completed items gives one a feeling of accomplishment. Performing priority items during prime time also assists in the best use and conservation of energy. The major benefit of managing time in this way is that it reduces stress by listing tasks and recording their accomplishment. At the end of each day, there is clear evidence of achievement.

Greater personal control over one's time provides greater work freedom. Time is not a renewable energy source; once lost it can never be regained. It is therefore critical that activities be planned to allow a balance of time between structured vs. unstructured activities. The following suggestions provide a means of gaining control over time in order to allow a balance between work and play.

Telephone Communication Techniques

- Have your objectives clearly in mind before you place a call.
- Give full attention to the person speaking.
- Summarize to keep the discussion moving.
- Use lunch or after-work time for less pressured social communication with people.
- Group telephone calls at one or two times during the day.
- Place your calls in priority order.
- Save time by being prepared before you place a call with the information you think may be required.
- Cut off the conversation at the point you perceive diminishing returns.

Meetings

To make meetings productive, the following will save substantial time:

- Establish a beginning and ending time.
- Always start on time; otherwise it reinforces late behavior.
- The last person to the meeting must take legible minutes and submit to chairperson after the meeting.
- Always establish a meeting agenda with items organized by priority and with estimated times for each item.

Tickler File

A simple technique developed in the early 1900s will not only keep your desk clear, but assist in planning and pacing your work. A "tickler file" involves about four to six inches of a file cabinet and includes 43 labeled folders. There is one folder for each month (12) and one for each day of the month (31).

- Start each day by taking out a folder for that day's activities.
- Every day that a task comes up place it in the appropriate month and/or day file for that day's "to-do" list.
- If other people need to be contacted, it is helpful to note in the folder where they can be reached and the appropriate phone number.
- Write on each month's folder those activities that occur consistently in the same month each year. Add suggestions for the following year.
- It is often helpful to establish both school and home tickler files.

Tape Recorders

- Use a tape recorder to clarify class rules, expectations and other appropriate information for substitutes, new students, or aides.
- A tape recorder can also provide personalized feedback in the form of personalized messages to students. These messages can be recorded during time traveling to and from school. At the end of the first message, provide an instruction for the student to summon the next student, e.g., "Please call Mary S. for her message. Thank you. Have a pleasant day."

Other Time Management Techniques

- Keep a clock in full view of yourself and visitors.
- Set up a "double cut-off time" so that if the first deadline is passed there will be an automatic second reminder.
- Keep your desk top cleared for work on the current piece of paper.
- Train subordinates to submit a recommendation along with a problem statement.

- Never put off for tomorrow what you can get someone else to do today.
- Learn to say no to requests.
- Maintain a small notebook for ideas.
- Remember the Pareto rule: Twenty percent of your work time achieves 80 percent of your work or, eighty percent of your time accomplishes only 20 percent of your work.
- Set goals and establish deadlines by making a daily "to do" list of items in order of importance.
- Make productive use of early morning work hours. This is a time of minimum interruptions.
- Get absolute "musts" completed first thing in the morning when your energy level is highest to avoid a crisis later in the day.
- Plan your day so that the important things get completed, recognizing that unpredictable events may limit some of your planned file time. The basic premise of time management assumes that one cannot do everything there is to do.
- Read professional publications as if they were newspapers by skimming for main ideas.
- Save routine tasks for the end of the day when you are tired.
- Keep a sheet of paper taped across the top of your TV. Log in how much time you watch TV each week. Ration yourself X hours of time per week. Use the time saved for something to accomplish, a high priority work or play activity.

Use of Leisure Time

Free time should be jealously guarded. Everyone periodically needs a totally free evening or weekend to just let go and not worry about gardening, projects, volunteer work, or other typical leisure-time consumers. One of the greatest gifts a person can give to him- or herself is a free time activity. Examples include strolling through the woods, a visit to a museum, or a trip to the library. Some other suggestions are shopping leisurely after work or simply going to the park to feed the squirrels. And doing something *new* from time to time, alone or with others, is highly recommended.

Maslach (1977) suggests a "decompression routine" of being alone for a while between leaving work and arriving home. Taking the scenic route home, turning the radio up, singing along, or just focusing on breathing can be individual methods of "decompressing." Other methods include forgetting work at dinner time and refraining from talking about the day's stressors.

Work-related professional conferences can be of more benefit when one can mix business with pleasure by going to dinner with a colleague or to lunch with an interested friend.

Time for Griping or Sharing

Griping and sharing are very different functions. Griping is counterproductive if practiced on a regular basis. One can easily waste an excessive amount of time griping rather than problem solving. However, it can be therapeutic to set scheduled sharing periods with an empathic friend. Make an appointment for a sharing session with an individual who will understand. Once a week or less should suffice as a designated "sharing time." Expressing personal concerns in a congenial setting rekindles pride and self-esteem.

If a group of colleagues meets on a regular basis, a short time allowance for "Ain't it Awful" should be established. When the time is up, the meeting should move on to more constructive subjects. If somebody breaks the rule, he or she should be required to buy a glass of wine or a cup of coffee for everyone.

Diary of Stress

Creative use of a small, spiral-type diary can help promote awareness and change stressful perceptions. Keeping an accurate diary of reactions to stress for a period of six weeks can help a person realize that one is often a poor observer of his or her own behavior. Unpleasant episodes or undesirable behaviors are often forgotten if not written down. It is not uncommon to fit partial recollections into a biased belief system. A diary helps to keep events relatively objective and fresh in memory.

It can be helpful to write in the left-hand column of the diary a brief description of events and a note about the strongest distress incident within each event. In the right-hand column indicate what preceded the event and what inner thoughts occurred before, during, and after the stressful event. Record the environment (people, places, and things) that surrounded the event. If one or more particular people stand out, underline their names. After a week of note taking, the observations should be reviewed, with emphasis upon patterns of conditions, people, and environments. What was thought or said to oneself (self-talk) should be carefully reviewed throughout each episode. A diary provides historic personal information otherwise impossible to reconstruct. It can be a powerful tool for awareness and self-change.

More Effective Discipline

According to Alschuler and Shea (1974), discipline is a constant struggle between teachers and students which occupies at least half of class time. Time spent on discipline is time which cannot be devoted to instruction. In order to learn, students must be attentive. On the average, students give their attention about half of a normal class period. Alschuler and Shea have contended that the battle for attention can become a contest between teacher and students. The plays include bantering, body language, ignoring, tone modulating, ordering, invoking, sarcasm, threatening, physical contact, refusing, complaining, escaping, intruding, and more.

Researchers have consistently concluded that the genesis of disciplinary action is a result of dysfunctional social relationships between teachers and students based upon inoperative rules and procedures. Student attention can be improved by determining when behavior problems specifically begin and which techniques are working or not working, by providing teacher training, and by clearly defining teacher role and responsibility.

In order to alleviate discipline problems, the following strategies have been found to be effective: identifying behavior, not getting hooked into game playing, pacing, increasing learning time, making individual teachers accountable, and using concerted school programs such as assertive discipline. One study reported by Alschuler and Shea found a 60 percent decrease in discipline referrals when a rumor was circulated that tenure, merit pay, and promotion were inversely tied to referrals.

The following is a quick checklist.

- Does every student understand the behavior I expect in my classroom?
- Do I ever threaten students without carrying through a punishment?
- Do I employ a planned, specific disciplinary system when a student misbehaves?
- Do the students clearly understand this system?
- Do I know what to do when a student initially misbehaves?
- Do I have an immediate method of dealing with a student who continues to misbehave?
- Am I consistent and fair in administering disciplinary actions?
- Do I have a planned positive reward system for identified positive behaviors?
- Do the students understand this reward system?

- Do I contact parents by phone or memo to discuss or review the expected behaviors and consequences prior to or at the beginning of each school year?
- Do I solicit suggestions from parents?
- Do I have a consistent policy for school work that is not turned in on time?
- Do I understand the resources of the school, and work in cooperation with other staff, and am I consistent with the total staff?
- Is there an isolation space for students who need to be temporarily alone?
- Do I have techniques for transition from one activity to another (a time when most misbehavior occurs)? Use of rotating student traffic directors or sustained silent reading is helpful.
- Do I have a system of non-verbal signals that students understand and that assist in self-control?

Huge (1981) described a five-step process of dealing with the most serious behavior problems. This process has successfully improved the deportment of 83 percent of the offending students. It includes:

1. While away from school, list the specific behaviors of one student that bother you most often. Be certain they are specific behaviors.
2. Schedule a conference with this difficult student away from the rest of the class. If necessary, ask someone to cover your class while you meet with the student.
3. Include in the conference the following:
   a. A statement by you as teacher indicating that the student is surely aware that there are certain behaviors on the student's part that are unacceptable to you as teacher. Then indicate these specific behaviors to the student.
   b. If you are comfortable, indicate to the student that because those behaviors irritate you, you then respond in a way that gets to the student. Give the student a chance to respond. Usually, he or she will simply say, "Yes, that's right."
   c. Then say, "When I'm upset because of these behaviors, I don't teach as well. When you get upset because of my reaction, you don't learn as well. Therefore, we're not going to do that any more. We're going to build a new plan."
4. Tell the student that from now on, whenever he or she is engaged in the specific behaviors that you have identified, you will indicate this by some non-verbal signal, such as eye contact, eye contact combined with scratching the head, touching on the

shoulder, etc. This non-verbal cue tells the student "You're doing it again, please stop." The student's responsibility is to keep score, by indicating on a 3" by 5" card or a sheet of paper every time the teacher gives the non-verbal signal. The student is to stop his or her behavior and put a mark on the paper or card. You assume through the entire process that the student will indeed stop every time you give the signal.

5. Post conference: Following the time segment that you have set aside to use the new plan (usually 30–40 minutes initially), you then meet with the student to receive his or her report to you regarding the number of times that you have had to give the non-verbal signal. In this conference, you must keep your patience regardless of how many times you've had to use the signal and tell the student, "Nice going. You did exactly what I wanted you to do. You stopped every time I gave the non-verbal signal. But the number of times we had to do it today was too many. Tomorrow it will be half that number. The next day, half of that. The next day none."

Time Out

A "time out" is an opportunity to take a short break from difficult school work, to relax, or to take a breather from a distressful activity in order to attend to another task. For example, if people-contact is excessive, a switch to paper work or reports offers a welcome change. It is sometimes helpful to exchange classes with a colleague for a day or make shifts in one's role to provide more variety. A time out for professionals who deal with dysfunctional people on a regular basis would be an opportunity to spend time with well-functioning, healthy people.

Preferred Activities

Engage in at least one preferred activity each day. For example, teachers might do a favorite art or science project. If administering, a principal might observe a master teacher, ask a supportive parent to lunch, or give an award to a deserving student. Preferred activities increase the likelihood of a pleasant and positive experience happening each day. Schedule such preferences immediately after a disliked activity. This makes even the most unpleasant of tasks more palatable when a payoff immediately follows.

Waiting

If one assumes the proper mental attitude, frustrations and liabilities can be turned into creative, constructive assets. If waiting is necessary, it might be considered a gift of time. Waiting can be turned into an opportunity rather than an inconvenience. It can be an experience of relaxation, mental diversion, or quiet planning.

Accepting What One Cannot Change

The past cannot be reconstructed. As Dale Carnegie (1944) said, "You can't saw sawdust . . . and . . . you can't go back and change dinosaur tracks [180 million years ago] . . . any more than you can change the words you uttered 180 seconds ago" (p. 93).

It is important to recognize and accept changes that are realistic and feasible. If a problem is beyond one's control, that fact should be accepted. Worrying about it simply wastes energy and adds to frustration. (One needs to allow for three or four really bad days per year, when everything may go wrong.) This familiar invocation says it all: "God grant me the serenity to accept the things I cannot change; the courage to change the things I can; and the wisdom to know the difference" (attributed to Reinhold Niebuhr, in Carnegie, 1944, p. 85).

PERSONAL PRESCRIPTIONS
FOR OCCUPATIONAL FEEDBACK/COMMUNICATION DEFICITS

Communication

Communication offers the possibility of being a major source of distress or a major solution to problems. Communication is a learned skill; consequently, some individuals are eloquent and others clumsy in their use of language. To be an effective communicator, one must first be confident and comfortable within oneself. Self-esteem means acceptance of one's own strengths and weaknesses. Being sensitive to the needs of others assists the communication process. Adapting to each individual, organizing information, explaining with clarity, detail, and ease, prevent distress. Also, learning to listen by interpreting, understanding, and responding in a way that verifies concern enhances the continuance of positive dialogue.

Some managers have developed the communication skill of making others feel at ease even when the content is potentially stressful. Communication can be punitive or rewarding. If punitive, it promotes fear or anger; if rewarding, it is likely to be enjoyed and anticipated. Albrecht (1979) enumerates a number of punishing and rewarding communications that need to be reviewed by individuals on a regular basis (see table 3).

By reviewing these lists, one can better determine his or her own style of communication. It is important to reflect upon how frequently one is sought out for information, sharing, or general conversation. Use of sensitive communication techniques discourages negative relationships. A rewarding style of communication will keep stress levels at a minimum and make life richer, as well as more enjoyable. One of the highest compliments that can be paid to an individual is to be called an effective communicator.

Telephone Calls

Keep a log of telephone calls both at home and at work. Record who, what, when, and why. Note the length of the call. Analyzing phone calls will assist in determining problem communication or callers. It takes little time to jot down this information and ultimately it is time-effective. As you become more aware of your telephone behavior, it will become easier to terminate unproductive calls or not respond yourself to some calls through delegation and more prudent decision making. Time management consultants have suggested that long-winded conversations can be terminated by remaining silent or tapping the button and indicating the signal is another call.

PERSONAL PRESCRIPTIONS
FOR WORK OVERLOAD

Organization of Priorities

Work overload usually occurs as a result of having too much to do in too little time. It is indigenous to education. Overload becomes defeating because it disrupts efforts toward organization of activities. It is more efficient to set aside enough time to complete one job and then move on to the next activity. It becomes very difficult to tackle one task at a time if one is overwhelmed by multiple projects each with its own pressing deadline.

By identifying roles and tasks, and assigning individuals on the basis of strengths, overload can be prevented. Establishing reasonable

TABLE 3

PUNISHING AND REWARDING COMMUNICATIONS

Punishing Communication	Rewarding Communication
Monopolizing communication	Giving others a chance to express or share information
Constant interruptions	Listening attentively
Showing disinterest or apathy	Sharing oneself
Withholding positive social cues (greeting, nods, eye contact)	Smiling/greeting/providing feedback
Using verbal abuse, barbs, or insults	Praising and complimenting
Using nonverbal put downs	Expressing respect for ideas or opinions
Complaining or whining	Giving suggestions constructively
Criticizing, ridiculing, or fault finding	Talking positively and supportively
Demanding and refusing to negotiate/compromise	Compromising and negotiating
Making others feel guilty/blaming/accusing	Affirming feelings and needs of others
Patronizing or talking down to others	Treating others as equals
Soliciting constant approval	Stating things honestly and sincerely
Losing one's temper frequently	Delaying emotional outbursts
Manipulating or being dishonest	Leveling with others by sharing information
Using "gotcha" or embarrassing others	Confronting others constructively
Telling lies, evading, or refusing to level with others	Staying on the conversational topic
Pushing others and overusing should/must/why	Agreeing with others when possible
Displaying frustration frequently	Asking straightforward, honest questions
Diverting conversation	Keeping the confidence of others
Playing with pencils, keys, coins, or fidgeting that diverts conversation	Being aware of nervous activities and recognizing communication stress symptoms
Inappropriate jokes	Joking and using good humor constructively
Insincere flattery or boasting too much	Expressing humility
Breaking confidences or failing to keep promises	Expressing genuine interest in others
Asking loaded or accusing questions	Gently asking sensitive questions

Note: Reprinted by permission from *Stress and the Manager* (pp. 265–267), by Karl Albrecht, © 1979, Prentice-Hall, Inc. Published by Prentice-Hall, Inc., Englewood Cliffs, N.J. 07632.

time limits and goals avoids overcommitment. It is sometimes necessary to eliminate lesser priority items for those of higher priority (i.e., based on the agreement of your supervisor). Individuals need to evaluate their most productive working time. For example, if they accomplish the majority of tasks in the morning, they should schedule the most difficult and highest priority items before noon.

Paper Work

As little paper work should be generated as feasible. Whenever possible, junk mail, memos, and other unnecessary paper should be thrown away. Ideally, a piece of paper should be handled only once. Eighty percent of what crosses a desk should be directed to the waste basket. This will leave full attention for the 20 percent that deserves productive response.

One time-saving idea is to keep on hand a set of pocket index cards upon which to summarize ideas found on many sheets of papers. Also keeping three file folders labeled "Today," "Pending/Future," and "Ongoing Projects" eliminates a myriad of paper scraps.

Compartmentalizing

Sir William Osler, the famous physician who organized the renowned Johns Hopkins School of Medicine, attributed his success to what he described as "day-tight compartments." He was inspired by this thought while voyaging on a luxury liner. The ship's metal doors could instantly close off various parts of the vessel into watertight compartments. Osler suggested (Carnegie, 1944) that one can avoid anxiety for tomorrow by pushing a button and hearing at every level of one's life the iron doors shutting out the past. He recommended that one should "let the dead past bury its dead. The load of tomorrow, added to that of yesterday carried today make the strongest falter. Shut off the future as tightly as the past" (p. 2).

Work should be left in the classroom or at the office when possible. If it absolutely must be taken home, the work should be done early to allow time for your mind to unwind and forget the difficulties of the day. On a tough day that has presented unresolved issues, it is wise to talk to a colleague, spouse, or close friend, then come to some decision. One should not let problems or unfinished tasks harbor or swell inside. Once school has been left behind, it should be forgotten. The following Sanskrit proverb succinctly summarizes compartmentalizing: "Yesterday is already a dream and tomorrow is only a vision, but today well lived makes every yesterday a dream of happiness and every tomorrow a vision of hope."

Looking Forward to Things

Sometimes when teachers or administrators are under distress because of work load, they tend to punish themselves out of subconscious guilt. Instead of reacting to guilt, however, it would be better to provide a reward for oneself. To keep spirits high it helps to look forward to a trip, dinner with a close friend, a show, a sports event, or some other treat. One should do something that has been a secret desire, such as learning to fly, sing, or participate in a campaign. When an individual feels good about him- or herself and involvement in outside activities, these positive feelings will be reflected at school.

On a visit to a special place it can be fun to take photographs, make tape recordings, or make notations in a diary. Hang the enlarged prints in the classroom or office. When things at work become pressured, focus on the pictures, recordings, or notes of this exhilarating experience. These will serve as a temporary diversion. The memory of pleasant associations can help take one's attention from the immediate stress.

When things get tedious, it is often helpful to throw oneself into a new and enjoyable project. A take-a-student (or parent) -to-lunch program where everyone can brown-bag it in a comfortable, natural setting is one such activity, easily instituted. An inservice session featuring a guest lecturer who deals with something fun and exciting can be planned, or there can be a periodic meeting to share funny stories or jokes. Some humor and informality can be built into scheduled meetings.

An hour a day might be set aside when no phone calls will be received.

Sensible Distractions

For many, learning how to play is the most difficult of all objectives. The workaholic educator can seldom be totally free of school work, nor can the person so wrapped up in work responsibilities that he or she doesn't take time for play. The pressures of school or family are more effectively dealt with when one can get away from them for a while. People who don't play are often irritable or depressed. Some people reward themselves with play time after a work accomplishment. Play is a necessary and important diversion from work.

If work becomes stressful, satisfaction can be obtained from sensible distractions that take one's mind off school. A hobby such as building, repairing, collecting, reading, or doing something totally different from educational activities provides a means of mental and physical rest. Doing something special with a child or getting a pet might be beneficial. When either fatigue or interruption prevents one from completing tasks, it is better to use sensible distractions.

The noted American psychologist William James gave an illustration of such a distraction. He said, "You know how it is when you try to recollect a forgotten name. Usually you help the recall by working at it, but sometimes the effort fails . . . and then the opposite expedient succeeds. Give up the effort entirely: think of something different, and in half an hour the last name comes sauntering into your mind, as Emerson says, as carelessly as if it had never been invited." By taking a mental break and substituting a sensible distraction, a person can later go back to work with renewed strength, vigor, and fervor. A demand made on the muscles instead of the gray matter not only gives the brain a rest but helps avoid frustration, as well.

Following is a brief checklist of sensible distractions:

Rest/naps
Games/sports/hobbies/hot tubbing
Hugging/holding/sharing
Meditation/prayer/quiet thought
Crying/reminiscing
Cultural/family traditions
Shopping/browsing
Jokes/laughter
Music/dancing/singing
Poetry/prose/leisure reading/book store/library
Nature/woods/beach
Museum/zoo/park
Puttering/idle play

Mental Diversions

Similar to sensible distractions are mental diversions. Individuals frequently set themselves up for anxiety by anticipating a highly stressful situation. For example, an upcoming speech, sports contest, or report usually involves reviewing and intensely focusing mental attention on the event. If a stressful telephone call is expected, a person may become jumpy, pace the floor, and be unable to take his or her mind off it. Frequently, these types of behavior lead to poorer performance.

By allowing yourself to indulge in a totally different mental activity, you might become more confident and less fearful. Spending a few minutes thinking of a positive situation (fishing, singing, walking in the woods, the ocean, a hobby) will occupy the mind with pleasure and displace worry and fear. This type of diversion confirms the knowledge that everything is relative after all. The author is reminded of an old saying, "I had the blues because I had no shoes, until upon the street I met a man who had no feet."

Everyone is on a terminal voyage; no one will live forever. Stress is part of the aging process. If stress is not controlled, it can speed the process of death. As mentioned in an earlier chapter, the Chinese define stress as both opportunity and danger. Individuals should avoid backing away from the opportunities or challenges of stress, yet not fall prey to the concomitant danger. By choosing how one intends to live, one can avoid the unnecessary waste of energy on distress. Being considerate of oneself will result not only in a much better quality of existence, but it may also extend life itself.

PERSONAL PRESCRIPTIONS
FOR CONTACT OVERLOAD

Skills in Communicating with Difficult People

Educators have little control over the people with whom they have contact each day. Philosopher Marcus Aurelius said, "I am going to meet people today who talk too much—people who are selfish, egotistical, ungrateful. But, I won't be surprised or disturbed for I couldn't imagine a world without such people."

In a similar vein, Abraham Lincoln had this to say, "All of us are the children of condition, of circumstances, of environment, of education, of acquired habits, and of heredity molding men as they are and will forever be."

In order to be successful in the field of education, it is necessary to have the skills and understanding to be able to deal with difficult people. It is important to be aware that different communication styles are required in dealing with various types of difficult personalities. Learning to communicate in ways that do not induce distress yet resolve conflicts is a necessity. Various communication techniques and courses are available to facilitate skills for communicating with obviously aggressive, passively resistant, affected, physically violent, highly dependent, or noncommittal type personalities.

Anger

Anger is both natural and necessary. It is perhaps the most common immediate response to frustration. It can be directed inwardly or outwardly. In reasonable doses it can provide relief and resolve situations. If excessive and non-directed, anger can be destructive.

One author (Greenberg, 1980) describes anger as a cover-up feeling for deeper hurt. It frequently covers this pain or hurt so effectively that one is not aware of the underlying feeling. Anger is thus an ego defense against more intense inner feelings. This inner hurt can be: rejection, fear, inadequacy, confusion, helplessness, uselessness, humiliation, despair, injustice, guilt, or insecurity.

If anger is a cover-up of more intense pain, it is important to accept anger as necessary and natural. If anger over a particular situation or person persists, deal with it after you have calmed down. Seek the underlying pain or hurt.

Most individuals who understand the underlying hurt become more able to control anger in future situations. Frequently the awareness of the underlying feeling (e.g., guilt) provides problem identification and possible solution. Awareness also makes one better able to understand and deal more effectively with anger.

Detached Concern

Lief and Fox (1963) first conceptualized the term "detached concern." They recognized that a certain amount of detachment was necessary in order to provide objectivity and healthy emotional distance from clients. Treating one's clients in a more objective and slightly more remote way permits less psychological discomfort and more effective service (Maslach, 1977).

A certain amount of empathy permits the development of mutual understanding and attachment between educator and client. The resulting relationship helps to foster mutual growth. However, it can also develop into a relationship of dependency or extreme distance. Educators are seldom formally trained to deal from a perspective of detached concern. Thus many are unable to maintain empathy, objectivity, and a healthy distance. Instead, they often rush in with enthusiasm and become too emotionally involved with their clients. Later, as a defense, when the helping process becomes overwhelmingly distressful, educators may become more calloused and insensitive. A healthy balance of emotion, involvement, and mutual respect is necessary between educators and the recipients of service.

Improved Interaction

It is very important that teachers and school administrators be aware of people with whom they work, and get to know them well. Once trust is established, they can mutually share thoughts and feelings. If possible, co-workers should have contact with each other at lunch, after work, or at social gatherings, getting to know as many people as possible within the school setting. Social contact provides a support system that is necessary for everyone. It is beneficial to let others know that they have been noticed and that they are considered worthwhile people. It is likewise important to be cooperative and honest with others. Sincerity is the foundation of close relationships. One should never be afraid to compliment or accept compliments from others.

In order to build relationships, an educator might start with one special co-worker or colleague. Then, if possible, gain two or three additional close school-related friends, making contact with them at least several times a week to discuss feelings and concerns about work and personal life. If mutual trust and respect, confidentiality, reciprocity, honesty, and sharing are evident, then most subjects can be discussed.

Social contact directly reduces stress by providing comfort and emotional support. If contact is made on a regular basis, the teacher should also be able to share ideas and solve problems with his or her principal. Although the teacher may find it difficult to share intimate information with the principal, the relationship can usually be mutually supportive. When it is necessary to discuss sensitive areas, another person can be found.

If close contacts at school are impossible to establish, educators might change departments or jobs, find a professional counselor, or socialize as much as possible with people outside the immediate work environment. Under any circumstances, one should gain a few real friends with whom to share the details of his or her life, rather than develop acquaintances with whom only superficial conversation and formal niceties are exchanged.

Appropriate Helping Roles

Educators want to help others; sometimes, without thinking, they offer unsolicited assistance. Some of these professionals assume at times that they know others' problems and have a ready answer. Instead of asking what clients need and guiding the clients to help themselves, educators sometimes use "rescue" techniques. Rescuing ultimately robs individuals of their self-respect and problem-solving skills. Providing unnecessary assistance to people who are capable of helping themselves is detrimental to both provider and receiver. It has been clearly documented that professionals burn out a great deal faster if they are constantly depleting their energy source by giving instead of guiding. Guidance involves assistance in problem identification and providing suggestions or opportunities for problem solving. Actual solutions should rest with the recipients of service. A good teacher or counselor provides support, reassurance, problem-solving opportunities, and practice for individuals to gain new coping techniques.

Concentration on Others

Sometimes, when distressed, a person may develop a pattern of excessive self-focus. When this begins to happen, it is wise to exert an extra effort to concentrate on others. Not only will it take the mind off one's own problems, it also will build friendships and provide inner satisfaction.

Hans Selye (1974) has described "altruistic egotism" as the selfish hoarding of goodwill, respect, esteem, support, and love of one's neighbor. He has perceived it to be the most efficient way to vent pent-up energy and to create enjoyable experiences, that is, being selfish in a way that will do a person the most good in the long run. People can assure their own happiness by accumulating the treasure of others' benevolence.

Philosophers and religious leaders for thousands of years have emphasized that if people love their neighbors as themselves, our world will be peaceful and loving. Aristotle called the same phenomenon "enlightened selfishness," or the joy of doing good for others which increases one's own health and happiness. Benjamin Franklin summed it up by saying, "When you are good to others, you are best to yourself. By thinking and concentrating on others, it avoids focus on one's own worries." Samuel Taylor Coleridge said, "The happiness of life is made up of the little charities of a kiss or smile, a kind look, a heartfelt compliment."

Education is a "people" profession, and most educators come into contact with many people each day. In order to make those contacts mutually beneficial, it is advisable to look for something pleasant in each association and to focus on the positive aspects of human interaction.

Humor

Norman Cousins, editor of the *Saturday Review*, reported using humor to cure a serious and painful disease (1977). For thousands of years people have been able to relieve stress by stepping back and laughing—at themselves, at others, or at situations. We have all experienced the easing of a tense situation by the right joke. Recognizing and using the elements of humor can make the most serious episode more palatable and less threatening. One of the most healthy types of humor is the ability to laugh at oneself. Most of us know that trauma is resolved when, after a harrowing experience, we can look back at it and find humor in it. Everyone has experienced pain, humiliation or fear which in retrospect can now cause a burst of mirth.

PERSONAL PRESCRIPTIONS
FOR ROLE CONFLICT/AMBIGUITY

Prevention of Role Conflict/Ambiguity

Role conflict arises when there is evidence of divergent expectations of an individual's job performance. It can be illustrated by the conflict which arises when a teacher, anxious to implement the school board's strict new homework policy, assigns a 200-word composition. The next morning an irate father calls to report that after participating in the school's spring concert, his daughter had to stay up beyond normal bedtime to complete the homework.

Role conflict is thus caused by pressures stemming from the opposing expectations of two or more individuals or groups. Role ambiguity, on the other hand, is the result of a lack of clarity about the extent of one's job. Role ambiguity is seen in the example of a principal who doesn't know whether she has the authority to send home a substitute teacher who appears to be under the influence of drugs or alcohol. Role conflict/ambiguity may be prevented or reduced by establishing clear role statements for each position.

Should the possibility exist that more than one supervisor will evaluate job performance, there should be joint determination beforehand of the performance goals selected for evaluation. Mutual understanding between supervisors and employee as to requirements should reduce the probability that the employee will be caught between conflicting expectations. Reviewing possible conflicts and ambiguities with the supervisor(s) avoids the likelihood of piecemeal work or crisis decision making. If unexpected role conflict or ambiguity develops, it should be addressed at the first sign of its existence. It is vital that problems be identified and addressed immediately for the benefit of both the organization and the individual, since role conflict/ambiguity can be crippling.

Resolution of Troubled Situations

Upon identification of a problem related to role requirements, supervisors and employees should move at once to find a solution. If conflicting expectations exist, something should be done immediately to make them consistent. Individuals should divest themselves of relationships that are draining or non-productive. They should take action to improve situations that are disconcerting, for example, revitalize work relationships or a marriage that has suffered from distress.

Troublesome work conditions should be discussed with supervisors and colleagues from a problem-solving standpoint. Difficult situations should not be left unresolved. One should surround oneself with positive thoughts, positive conditions, and positive people. The establishment of rewarding, pleasant, cooperative relationships with people can help one to avoid troubled circumstances.

Development of Diplomatic Assertiveness

In a conflict, it is very easy to allow oneself to become either passive or abusive. To act in a diplomatic, yet assertive manner is a skill few possess. Diplomacy simply means recognition that other people need self-respect. The desirable quality of being direct and honest needs to be balanced with sensitivity to others. Saying things in the most sincere, yet direct way will make both parties retain respect and confidence in themselves and in one another.

From time to time, everyone experiences anger and frustration. Taking time to sort out feelings and understanding the potential consequence of energy-robbing explosions can help resolve problems rather than intensify them. Taking responsibility for feelings by using "I" rather than "You" is another means of making feelings clear, direct, and honest. In problem resolution, it is beneficial to express what is desired from the person upon whom the anger is focused.

Resistance

Key factors in reducing role conflict are awareness and resolve to overcome personal resistance. As is the case in the physical sciences, resistance to others or to change may only negate another energy force. Shakespeare wrote, "Heat not a furnace for your foe so hot that it do singe yourself." The result of blind resistance is apt to be a firmly established power struggle; combining forces provides unity and momentum, and often yields successful solutions. Compromise through discovery of common purposes and development of mutual understanding are frequently desirable. Individuals and work groups often focus on their differences; instead, they should discover and build on their common interests and needs. This approach requires that individuals be open to new ideas and give them serious consideration. It does not imply abdication of principle. Cooperation frequently becomes contagious and brings about a chain reaction which may result in higher group morale as well as individual self-esteem.

Conservation of Energy

Wasting psychological energy adds to burnout. Energy should be guarded as a valuable commodity. As mentioned earlier in this chapter, a diary might be used to record the activities which use energy during the course of each day. One should reserve sufficient energy for those tasks and outside activities that bring the most satisfaction. Burning off energy through frustration, anger, or pointless activity is counter-productive. Replenishment of energy can occur more sensibly if a fulfilling life exists both inside and outside the classroom or school office.

Maintenance of Consistent Behavior Patterns

It is good to maintain a steady level of activity and productivity. Rapid changes in activity level appear to create conditions for distress. Such rapid swings also appear responsible for the high level of tension found among air traffic controllers, emergency room attendants, police, fire fighters, and other crisis intervention workers.

A person of any occupation or personality type who moves from calm to crisis on an unpredictable basis faces the possibility of eventual malfunction caused by the body's alarm reactions. Crisis intervention involves intense emotions. Insofar as it is possible, one should limit the frequency with which one is involved in major crisis intervention activities. A school administrator can delegate certain responsibilities and use available resources in a preventive manner so as to reduce the probability of having to resort to crisis intervention. Remaining relatively consistent in one's activity patterns is a measure that seems to contribute to longer life.

Dealing with Guilt or Worry

Frequently feeling guilty about not living up to someone else's ideal doesn't build good mental health. No one can hope to be perfect; a person is capable only of his or her best efforts. Worry does not undo a wrong or correct what has already gone awry.

Randomly reading from a history book will confirm that the world has always been in the throes of agony and tragedy. This fact should not be taken lightly, but worrying about it is not the solution either. Worrying can create a vicious circle—for instance, worrying about insomnia usually causes more damage through additional sleeplessness. This "distress of distress" is summed up in an old saying: "Remember, today is the tomorrow you worried about yesterday." Some great figures of history voiced their opinion about worry:

> *Pericles:* "Come, gentlemen, we sit too long on trifles."
> *Epictetus:* "There is only one way to happiness and that is to cease worrying about things which are beyond the power of our will."
> *Disraeli:* "Life is too short to be little."
> *George Bernard Shaw:* "The secret of being miserable is to have the leisure to bother about whether you are happy or not."

By keeping active, busy, enthusiastic, and interested in our work and in others, the possibility of worry decreases. Too often we waste energy on reactive worry rather than proactively seeking problem resolution.

One way to manage this form of stress is to construct a "worry list," writing down each worry and a proposed plan for dealing with it. By getting such concerns out in the open, one can more effectively review and resolve them. It might help to read a book like Dale Carnegie's *How to Stop Worrying and Start Living* (1944), or even Wayne Dyer's *Your Erroneous Zones!* (1976).

Control of Interruptions

Certain periods of each day should be scheduled for your own purposes. Setting aside 10–60 minutes of uninterruptable time daily—during which you are not available to receive phone calls or deal with the needs of others—will provide an opportunity to renew energies or to concentrate on completion of a project.

PRESCRIPTIONS REGARDING
INDIVIDUAL FACTORS

Strong Family Life

The late Lewis B. Terman, psychologist and dean at Stanford University, initiated the most comprehensive longitudinal study of individuals ever conducted (Goleman, 1980). Although his study focused only on highly intelligent individuals, his results can be generalized. More than 1,500 people were studied over a 60-year span. Terman's most significant finding was that a strong family life served as the best predictor of a successful and satisfying life. Although work was found to be important, good marital and family relations were most important to successful living. If one's family remains the top priority, satisfaction at work will be more likely and more stable. Positive family relations can buffer the effect of occupational stress. Home is regarded as the place where individuals can remove their masks and relieve stress. A family's love, respect, and understanding can relieve fear or worries and melt the tensions absorbed during a difficult day. Without the family for respite and renewal, the effects of distress could continue to gain momentum.

Memorabilia

Everyone feels melancholy periodically. If over the years one has saved letters, cards, thank you's, letters of recommendation, poems, quotes, personal notes, or other emotionally inspiring mementos, he or she has available a potent source of renewed optimism. Sifting fondly through mementos reawakens emotional inspiration. These remembrances usually provide an opportunity to forget current concerns and look forward to more pleasant events. Playing a favorite record or reviewing a collection of papers on positive mental health can also offer relief. For an occasional laugh, keeping a "Foolish Foibles Folder" of silly things we have done adds levity in the face of difficult chores.

Avoidance or Control of Drastic Changes

A move to a new city, a new job, or a new home can require a great deal of adjustment. If too many changes come within a short time, distress can more easily occur. In 1949, Thomas H. Holmes began giving systematic attention to the case histories of more than 5,000 patients (Holmes & Rahe, 1967). He found that a number of life-change events occurred repeatedly. These events tended to cluster over a brief time period just prior to the onset of a major illness (see the Holmes Scale in Appendix A). Major events that can cause distress are: a new or different job, divorce or marital separation, death of a close family member or close friend, marriage, sexual difficulties, new family member, major change in financial status, child leaving home, a large mortgage, difficulties at work or change in work status, and major personal habit change. Interestingly, Holmes also found positive stress events—such as the "instant" success of a writer or musician—can also cause distress. Avoiding or leaving space to accommodate these significant changes will decrease emotional wear and tear.

One can frequently exercise a large amount of individual control over the events of marriage, moving, going to college, or the addition of a family member. Some life changes cannot be avoided, but it would be advisable to avoid adding additional life changes during crisis periods. The ability to space significant events not only increases control, but also helps to prevent health problems.

Exercise

After a day of difficult work we owe our minds and bodies an opportunity to shake out the cobwebs. Exercise is an excellent way to burn off excess adrenalin that accumulates during a stressful day. Paradoxically, if one feels tired, exercise usually provides revival. Walking, swimming, jogging, playing tag football, or working out in a gym are helpful. The more enjoyable the activity and the more totally involved the participant becomes in the exercise, the more likelihood there is that life pressures can be controlled.

The major benefits of an exercise program include:

- developing an efficient cardiovascular system, thereby reducing the chance of heart disease;
- lowering blood pressure;
- relieving stress and muscle tension;
- controlling body fat;
- slowing the deterioration of bones;
- providing a sense of psychological, as well as physical, well-being.

Unhappily, more live by the myths of exercise than the realities. Consider some of the more common excuses: "There's no point in exercising because it increases my appetite." (Actually, exercise will reduce appetite, especially if it is undertaken just before mealtime.) "It takes six hours of bike riding or nine miles of jogging to lose a pound, and I simply don't have that kind of time," or "I'm too old to exercise," or "I get all the exercise I need at home." Each is an attempt at avoidance, frequently a result of limited or inaccurate information or established habits that do not include exercise.

One of the most physically demanding jobs is that of longshoreman. Yet a study of San Francisco dock workers reported by Schafer (1978) indicated that longshoremen were only half as likely to have heart attacks as men with less strenuous jobs.

The Madison, Wisconsin, school system instituted a full-scale physical fitness program for its 120-member management staff. They began in September 1978, when the school district persuaded its insurance carrier to pick up 62 percent of the program cost. Reports now indicate that the system is reaping the benefits of higher productivity and fewer health-related costs. Before the program started, the Madison school system had been disturbed by increased costs of insuring unhealthy employees: (1) workers' compensation costs increased by 176 percent in three years; (2) disability insurance increased by 46 percent in five years; (3) absenteeism increased 15 percent in four years; (4) health claim costs increased 286 percent in three years.

Once into the fitness effort, Madison administrators looked and felt better, and many reported significant changes in their life styles. The program began with a health appraisal. Over one-third had excessively high levels of cholesterol, one-quarter were dangerously overweight, one-half were not getting sufficient exercise, and almost 10 percent had blood pressure at the high-risk range. The program provided two major elements: exercise (running, swimming, bicycle riding) and education (relaxation exercises, weight control, attitude, diet). Very few administrators failed to participate in the program.

Other exercise suggestions include:

• Organize an after-school jogging, tennis, or badminton club.
• Keep exercise equipment in the school facility.
• Participate in swimming, sauna, handball, golf, tennis, or other active sports.
• If all else fails, take a short walk. It will keep your body refreshed and alert.

Individuals should not try to increase exercise activities too quickly, especially if over 35 years of age. Instead, each person should first get a physical examination and start with slow, progressive steps toward reconditioning. Begin with walking or slow jogging so that you can maintain the pace, and exercise becomes rewarding, not defeating. Instead of trying to prove that your physical shape can be regained instantly, take time and savor each new accomplishment. It is important to reward oneself for new vigor and attitude.

Rest and Relaxation

William James, America's first psychologist, observed, "Tension is a habit. Relaxation is a habit, and bad habits can be broken and good habits formed." The heart beats approximately 72 times every minute. During an average 70-year life span, the heart will beat two and one-half billion times. It will pump 100 million gallons of blood through 60,000 miles of blood vessels—enough to fill a 4,000 gallon tank each day. When beating at this rate, it is actually working nine hours out of 24. In the aggregate, its rest period totals a full 15 hours a day. The well-publicized "disastolic measurement" indicates pressure within an artery when it is relaxed between heartbeats.

The parasympathetic nervous system mitigates the fight-or-flight reaction by slowing the breath rate and heartbeat while lowering hormone flow and blood pressure. This reaction is the body's natural means of providing a rest cycle. In order for the body to remain in a healthy, responsive state, it automatically balances emergency activities with a rest phase. Rest provides for more efficient body functioning. All of us have experienced an occasional restless night, the subsequent inefficiency of the next day, and the body's need for more rest the next evening. When there is a disruption of the rest cycle, the body sends out ominous signals. Periods of rest and relaxation are appropriate responses to those signals—responses which, in fact, may be necessary for survival. It should be noted that periods of relaxation should be reasonably brief. An excess of relaxation can be as harmful as too much stress.

It is important to differentiate rest from relaxation techniques. Relaxation techniques are learned skills aimed at keeping the body at a consistent level of energy conservation. Rest periods are aimed at temporary removal from work or other stressful activities. A rest period can be a few minutes' break or a two-week vacation; it might involve reading a book, going hunting or fishing, visiting a friend, watching TV, going out to dinner, or walking in the park. Rest does not always conserve energy, nor is it necessarily a passive activity. Relaxation techniques are mind/body activities that can be used at any time to ameliorate the effects of regular stressors.

Nutrition

Nutrition is much more a function of personal life style than is generally realized. It is not just what, but how, why, and when you eat that matters.

How you eat is important. In general, it is wise to eat food that is easily digested and assimilated. Try to avoid the "eat and run" syndrome, stuffing yourself or gulping your food. Eating in a relaxed atmosphere and chewing food well are both factors which contribute to better digestion.

Where and when you eat should also be a consideration. It is wise to avoid eating late at night or when you are anxious and unable to eat slowly. Eating while moving, driving, standing or doing something else which demands attention at the same time is hard on your body's digestive process.

Awareness of why you eat is helpful. Ask yourself how often you eat because you are bored, anxious, feel social pressure, are tired, or need oral gratification. Try to distinguish these feelings from the sensation of hunger and avoid impulsive self-indulgence.

Be concerned with what you eat, but don't let worry about food take up too much of your energy. Most of us should consume more whole grains, cereals, fresh fruits and vegetables, fish, poultry, and legumes, and should investigate alternative protein sources. The dangers of too much sugar, salt, fat and cholesterol, food dyes and preservatives, alcohol, and caffeine are well known.

Eating is a daily behavior that plays an important role in all of our lives. It is better to think in terms of "eating to live" rather than "living to eat."

Moderation

The California Department of Public Health identified seven health practices that had very positive effects (Belloc, 1973). They are:

- Sleeping approximately seven hours per day.
- Eating breakfast every day.
- Not eating between meals.
- Not becoming seriously overweight.
- Participating in moderate physical activity.
- Not smoking.
- Drinking only moderate amounts of alcohol.

Perhaps the most significant word is moderation; this includes moderation in drink, food, physical activity, etc. Being reasonable about daily habits appears to produce positive results.

Avoidance of Unnecessary Medication

There are many chemicals that can mask the symptoms of stress. None of these chemicals actually enhances natural body adjustment to change. Many medications simply provide temporary, symptomatic relief by destroying pain or providing momentary euphoria or calm. Unfortunately, many drugs are habit forming (e.g., alcohol or mild tranquilizers). Often they result in a form of psychological flight that eventually causes more stress. By freeing oneself from dependence on drugs such as antacids, tranquilizers, or alcohol, one can then deal directly with the cause of distress. The ability to handle occupational stress lies within the individual and the organization, not in the use of drugs. Resolution of distress involves awareness, planning, and large doses of practice.

Sexual Activity

The role of sexual fulfillment as a tension reducer is often ignored. Sexual activity, like nuclear energy, can be a constructive release or a battleground of destruction. Life devoid of real love and concomitant physical contact is vacuous. The combination of a strong commitment and sexual fulfillment can significantly reduce the distress of life.

Insomnia Control

There are many degrees of insomnia. They vary from restless sleep, to periodic awakening, to not sleeping at all for lengths of time. Preventive techniques for insomnia include:

- Bedtime should not include or be preceded by serious thinking, TV, or paper work. These activities generally tend to overstimulate the mind and can create sleeping disturbances.
- Decrease or eliminate the use of stimulants such as coffee or tea. A glass of milk is a better alternative.
- If you have experienced a particularly distressful day, sit down in a quiet place (not the bedroom) and allow 10–15 minutes to reflect on a problem of the day. If a solution does not arrive, compliment yourself for understanding the symptoms of tension and decide to

take the problem up the next day when more information is available. Let go of the problem and move on to another relaxing activity prior to bed.

Insomnia intervention activities include:

- Don't allow more than about ten minutes to pass without falling asleep. If still awake, get up, go into a different room, and read, write, or perform a quiet, relaxing activity. Use relaxation exercises before retiring again.
- If awake, don't look at the clock to see what time it is; it only focuses further on the problem.
- Allow the mind to ruminate. Don't fight the flow of thoughts, let them pass. Think of a pleasurable activity or a single word or number.
- Relax through transcendental meditation, body awareness, and muscle relaxation.
- If insomnia continues for several weeks after using these techniques, see a counselor.

PRESCRIPTIONS
FOR TRAINING DEFICITS

Learning

Learning is the natural extension of consciousness and expansion of the mind. Reading a novel or learning about new places, things, or activities provides an opportunity to escape from the "all work and no play" syndrome. This type of learning also helps a person to become a better educator, as well as a well-rounded and better-informed person.

A first step could be to review your own job requirements and determine your areas of expertise or strength, as well as areas of need. After identifying the most positive attributes you bring to your job, rank your current work needs. Determine which major growth activities might enhance personal and job-related growth. If other workers have similar needs, convince the organization to provide workshops, conferences, or course work. If your personal growth needs are unique, enroll in a workshop or university course.

Be careful not to assume new obligations to a point where they overextend personal and work load capacities. Learning new ideas and methods directly related to one's work can be self-renewing, but in excess it can be destructive. If a class or other activity is too dull, too difficult, or not helpful, don't be afraid to withdraw from it rather than continue it in pain and frustration.

Commitment to Effort

Making a conscious effort to do one's best will bring about both internal and external rewards. This can be accomplished by keeping alert to changing methodologies and philosophies, attending periodic workshops and conferences, sharing with other staff members, keeping active with hobbies and outside interests, listening and responding to students, parents, and other professionals, and reading for recreation as well as for professional improvement. If a person is confident that he or she is doing his or her best, the criticisms of others will not adversely affect performance.

Abraham Lincoln expressed his concern about doing one's best. He said:

> If I were to try to read, much less to answer, all the attacks made on me, this shop might as well be closed for any other business. I do the very best I know how—the very best I can and I mean to keep on doing so until the end. If the end brings me out all right, then what is said against me won't matter. If the end brings me out wrong, then ten angels swearing I was right would make no difference.

Writing Goals

Writing can serve as a problem-solving technique. Sometimes by writing down problems, an individual can begin to resolve issues that have been ignored or found difficult. If a problem is determined to be insoluble, that in itself is a type of solution in that it brings closure to continued resolution efforts.

Goals should first be expressed clearly in writing and then divided into sequential elements that lend themselves to step-by-step attainment. The power of clear direction is immeasurable. Knowing what one wants and how to accomplish it through a logical method is far superior to expecting achievement through haphazard efforts. Systematic progress can best be achieved by first putting a written plan together.

Awareness of Strengths and Weaknesses

According to Gmelch (1977) and Page (1966), school administrators (like Caesar) try to be all things to all people. Instead, they must be reeducated in the art of measuring their own physical and psychological capabilities and limitations. As administrators identify their own particular strengths and weaknesses, they should examine their regular activities to see which are fun or frustrating, which are challenging or boring, and which lead to fulfillment or distress. Through this process, latent talents can be discovered and limitations can be unveiled. With heightened awareness, where capabilities are evident, one can focus on success, and improve or delegate in those areas where limitations are known.

Modeling

Coping with distress is a learned behavior, one which can be developed through observation, experience, and practice. Imitating another's coping behavior may appear simplistic; yet, imitation is how most of us learn any concept. Children, adolescents, and adults alike learn an extraordinary amount simply by observing and copying others. By imitating successful models, one can gain new coping techniques. Select a couple of tolerant, understanding, informed individuals with whom you can share mutual respect and who are willing to provide support. You should then study, rehearse, and continue to practice the coping behaviors of one or more models.

Rehearsal

If one feels stressed by a particular event, an excellent prescription is to reconstruct it and mentally rehearse a positive solution. Say aloud the names of the people, things, or activities that provide for the solution. Rehearse with a feeling of confidence and mastery. Practice the acts which are necessary to achieve the solution, and then employ them in the future. Plan how to respond to the next new challenge.

Establishing a Personal Contract

Recognizing the internal alarm bells that signal distress leads to the early identification of harmful stressors. Once a person decides to do something about the source of stress, he or she should act quickly. The longer one tolerates a distressful situation, the more difficult it will be to gain control over it.

It is now time to establish a realistic objective. Seek a solution—get needed advice and then write up a personal contract. Establish a means of measuring progress. It is best to use a step-by-step, goal-setting approach. Don't attempt too much at one time; start with small, achievable goals.

Many people have found that a personal contract co-signed by another is a useful method of making a commitment to managing stress. Involve a close friend or relative to help provide social support, encouragement, and to be a witness to the new undertaking. Such a contract might state: "I have agreed to begin a program of stress management and will start by utilizing . . . I will measure progress by . . . I will reevaluate . . . I will reward myself by . . . ."

SUMMARY

An individual can *learn* to cope with stress. There are many ways to prevent or lessen the negative effects of distress. Learning involves personal awareness, planning, practice, and persistence. The ability to withstand stress is dependent on both physical and emotional fitness. A strong body is aided by exercise, proper nutrition, and appropriate amounts of sleep and rest, as well as moderation in personal habits. A healthy mind includes a positive attitude toward self and others, realistic expectations, patience, a happy balance between work and play, knowing one's own strengths and weaknesses, good communication skills, variety of activities, conservation of energy, and a sense of personal control. Much more can be accomplished by approaching a known stressful situation as a challenge or opportunity rather than as a danger or threat. Potentially negative energy can be transformed into motivational and productive energy through personal resolution.

Utilizing the techniques in this chapter, which have been found to be situationally effective, can greatly aid an individual toward a healthy and productive life.

CHAPTER IX

Organizational Means
of Distress Reduction

Today, the United States is a society based on organizations. Less than a century ago, only 3 percent of the population worked for organizations. Now, nine out of ten people work for organizations. Education is, in fact, the largest generic organization in this country.

AN ORGANIZATIONAL PLAN

Every organization, no matter how small, needs to establish a plan for the safety and health of its employees. Although it is the responsibility of all organizational personnel to pursue such a plan, accountability lies with the governing board and top management. It is this group that guides the assignment of personnel and determines their well-being. It is also this group that acts as the prime mover for fostering constructive change. We no longer have the luxury of a simple world with small, personal organizations. We live in a highly complex, ever-expanding world of technological and social revolution. Similarly, school organizations of most large cities are equally vast and complex. In order to survive under these conditions, school systems must adapt their work practices to accomplish their goals and to provide for the well-being of employees.

Any plan to reduce organizational stress needs to take into account a number of factors. They include:

1. Appraisal of the current state of affairs of the school organization, including each job position. This appraisal would include

an investigation or survey of educator attitudes to gain baseline data on: current levels of satisfaction, health, levels of stress/distress, sources of stress/distress, quality of labor-management communication, degree of feedback to employees, and job analyses to evaluate work overload and role ambiguity.

2. Planning a program for stress reduction that involves school employees, is sequential, and addresses the major priorities established by the appraisal (no. 1 above). Employ outside professional assistance if necessary. Planning involves gaining and maintaining the participation of employees at every stage. Planning should also take into account costs, timeliness, master plan, and implementation. It has been suggested that the organization that fails to plan, plans to fail.

3. Implementation, or putting the plan into action, assumes readiness. It is important that every member of the organization be adequately prepared for the new program, even if its goal is to provide stress relief. Keep participation voluntary so that it is not a forced choice, but provides an individual option and ownership. Interestingly enough, the simplest plans and implementation design will fare the best. Elaborate plans may be too complex or cumbersome to implement. A formal implementation design will take into account the top one or two priorities only. Lower priority items may need only permission or encouragement for employees to undertake (e.g., physical fitness during lunch or after work).

An informal public relations and publicity campaign will help highlight implementation of the program to reduce organizational stress. But don't be surprised if there is some negativism or cynicism. The best laid plans can be sabotaged by a few. Some may look for hidden meanings or question the organization's trust or intent. Schools are often subject to scapegoat criticism, so some public outcry might be expected. Voltaire said, "Those who walk on the welltrodden path throw stones at those who are showing a new way." Galileo, Einstein, da Vinci, the Wright brothers, and many others were severely criticized for their attempts to make a better world for people.

4. Evaluation and reevaluation of the program make up the most important step of all. Unless there is periodic built-in reevaluation, all efforts are for naught. It is also important because initial perceptions can be the result of overenthusiasm and "halo effect," a bias based upon one's general impression or mind set.

Responsibility for reevaluation, like planning, should be shared by school administrators and school employee representatives. If each has a specific role in stress management, it will assist not only in reevaluation, but maintenance of a sound stress management program. Establish criteria for measuring the success of the program and assess these periodically. Also, appraise each program component on a regular basis to determine necessary course corrections. Revise the program as reevaluation data indicate and continue to make occupational health for employees the highest priority. Stress management is not only an organizational responsibility but a commitment to the organization's future.

Criteria Indicating the Quality of an Organizational Plan

There are many criteria that can be measured to indicate the success of a plan to reduce organizational stress. These include:

1. Employees are in good health, with the incidence of distress, disease, absenteeism, and job turnover at a practical minimum.
2. Employees feel that they and others are working toward a standard of excellence within the organization.
3. Employees express overall satisfaction with their work roles and feel they are continuing to move toward greater job satisfaction.
4. Employees have high morale and express positive relationships with peers, superiors, and subordinates. Rivalry is healthy, but work politics are negligible.
5. Employees strongly support the organization, its structure, policies, and goals and strive toward organizational objectives.
6. Employees work productively and effectively as defined in their job descriptions. They have a clear understanding of their roles and role relationships, as well as a shared commitment to identified organizational goals.
7. Employees tend to support change because they feel they have adequate participation in decisions that affect them.
8. Employees are well informed about the affairs and objectives of the organization. There are few negative rumors about members, policies, or procedures of the organization. There is a minimum of counter-productive cliques. There is little need, if any, for outside intervention.
9. Employees and their families participate in the social activities of the organization. Families feel good about the role and function of the employed member and the organization in general.
10. Employees receive regular feedback regarding their performance within the organization.

11. Managers are visible, real, accessible, sensitive, and approachable by all members of the organization. Management is continually aware of the status and needs of each department or subgroup.
12. Employees understand and feel they are all working for the same basic good—the continued strength and growth of the organization.
13. All levels of employees feel respected, loved, and an important part of the organization—like a healthy family where all members are valued and divisions of labor are based on individual strengths and abilities.

Another measure of an organization's health is its social climate (Albrecht, 1979). This may be expressed in terms of camaraderie, respect, and morale. With respect to social climate, there are at least three areas that need to be studied:

1. degree of employee identification with the organization;
2. extent of labor-management polarization;
3. employee's importance in the organization as perceived by those in higher positions.

The continuum of identification-alienation refers to the extent to which employees identify themselves with the organization—they either take pride, cooperate, and initiate positive membership in the organization, or they openly criticize, resist, or express apathy about their association with the organization. Employee attitude questionnaires or random survey samplings can assist in assessing this dimension. Managers can foster positive identification by simply recognizing and rewarding individual achievements. Newsletters and other communication/feedback devices are helpful in creating a positive, caring impression of the organization to its staff.

The continuum of labor-management polarization refers to the extent of distance expressed between "ruling" vs. "working" classes. The greater the distance, the larger are the difficulties related to productivity and job satisfaction. Managers and union leaders must take the initiative to foster better relations. One means is to make top and lower level managers more visible. Another is for management to listen to and use the ideas and suggestions of all employees. A third approach is to provide participative decision making. Good two-way communication is perhaps the strongest antidote to labor-management polarization.

Perceived importance in the organization refers to the amount of individual attention paid to employees. At one extreme, employees can feel like just a number; at the other end of the scale, the feeling of being valued may be positive and rewarding. The social climate of an organization determines these perceptions. If management relates personally to all levels of employees, they will have a feeling of importance. If, however, the majority of personal contact is reprimanding, disciplinary, or "just the facts," the results can be unproductive.

The use of surveys or informal chats can alert managers to the degree to which employees feel themselves to be valued. Constructive changes can be made, such as altering impersonal behaviors to personal ones, keeping communication channels open, and staying in close contact with all levels of staff.

The following organizational prescriptions for distress reduction are grouped in relation to the seven primary causes of occupational stress in education (for a full discussion of the seven causes, see Chapters III–V). Each potential solution activity was assigned to its assumed primary cause of distress. Although far from exhaustive, this plan will offer educators an attempt to rethink and reorganize their objectives, as well as their current practices. If today's educational enterprise is to continue to provide quality education, it may need significant reorganization.

ORGANIZATIONAL PRESCRIPTIONS
FOR IMPROVED CONTROL OVER ONE'S WORK DESTINY

Organizational Changes

The typical school district assigns 4–6 percent of its total staff to supervisory positions; industry commonly designates 12–25 percent (Cedoline, 1980). This means that three to four times the number of supervisory personnel are available in industry as compared to education. In the absence of proper supervision in the field of education, it is not surprising that public outcry for quality and accountability has increased. Industrial management studies clearly establish the ideal ratio of supervision to be 6–12 employees per full-time manager. The typical school principal supervises between 20 and 48 staff members.

Employees in every field need ongoing supervision and assistance if they are to be expected to perform quality work. This is no less true in education. Surveys of teachers with three or fewer years of service tend to verify their need for ongoing supervision and training. School administrators likewise need close guidance and supervision, especially at initial stages of their careers. Few, if any, major industrial corporations place a manager in a new position without intense follow-up training. Until the ratio of administrators to staff in public education becomes closer to that in industry, we will continue to hear negative outcry from the public regarding the quality of education.

Reassignments

When an employee is performing at less than desirable levels, every attempt should be made to provide appropriate assistance in those areas where improvement is needed. When unsatisfactory performance continues despite concentrated assistance over a reasonable period of time, career redirection should be considered. The employee needs either a change of occupation or a new work environment. It is the responsibility of the employer through management to provide these types of assistance.

Transfer or reassignment should not be reserved for the incompetent, nor should transfer be viewed as only negative and involuntary. Employees deserve the right to know that a transfer is being considered. Since involuntary transfer has been rated as the number one problem in at least two recent research studies (see Chapter III), it bears further attention by educators. Educational transfer policies should, as in industry, provide professional growth and be viewed as a positive, promotional experience. School districts might strongly consider reassignment as a positive, expected change every four or five years.

Salary

Organizations should carefully assess the concept of rewards for workers. The most obvious reward, money, is a basic necessity and should be respected as such. A decent salary is necessary to allow employees to live a balanced life. Public organizations often hire and maintain staff at very low salaries and postpone raises due to lack of funds.

Bryan (1981) reported that the tighter the funding, the higher the burnout rate will be for staff and others affiliated with the organization. He emphasized that when the issue of money is downplayed by management or not treated as a legitimate need, it can cause good employees to drop out or become disillusioned with their work.

Money is not the only possible reward but when all that remains is idealism, dedication, and commitment to the work ethic, one becomes vulnerable to burnout. Distress becomes more imminent when sixty-hour weeks, breakfast meetings, missed lunch breaks, and evening work go unnoticed and unrewarded. Organizations cannot maintain low salary standards and expect to contract or retain staff members simply for "the good of the cause." Reasonable compensation should be considered a top priority for any organization with concern for morale and productivity.

Fiscal Reorganization

Finance in education can be equated with the weather—both are unpredictable. Seldom does a school district know what its funding will be until near the opening of the academic year. Genuine reform in education cannot occur until a consistent fiscal base is established.

Most school district employees are paid on the basis of a schedule that provides a stepwise increment in salary based upon length of tenure. On the typical schedule, salary is not adjusted on the basis of performance. Employees are paid for the number of years of service (usually to a maximum level of 10–15 years), and frequently for the number of college courses taken and degrees acquired. The arrangement would appear bizarre to the average business person. Education provides few, if any, incentives for performance and little opportunity for promotion or recognition. It is not surprising that some educators become apathetic after 5–8 years in the profession. At that point motivation is usually based on purely intrinsic rewards (love of teaching, parent support, a child's smile, etc.). Fortunately there are many devoted, highly conscientious educators, or apathy would be epidemic. However, until performance is rewarded by salary recognition and advancement, motivation will be stifled.

Other Rewards for Performance

There is a need to provide recognition and rewards to educators for service or achievement in related areas. Energy conservation, for example, may be a major local priority. Teachers and administrators who accomplish significant energy cost savings might be rewarded with part of the savings. School staffs need to be part of local decision-making teams. Involvement in community activities should be "written in" to and consonant with the goals and objectives of the school board. There are many opportunities that can be used to support rather than dissipate energies. A reward need not be monetary; it may be recognition through a plaque, a local newspaper article, or an announcement at a public meeting.

Administrative Flextime

Flextime is a work scheduling system that allows employees to choose (within limits) their own hours. The practice has been spreading in American business, largely because workers have been pressing for it. Nearly half the companies adopting flextime have discovered an added bonus; according to a new survey, flextime seems to increase productivity through improved morale and lower absenteeism.

Since its debut in the early 1970s, an estimated 13 percent of all U.S. companies have adopted variants of the new system. Flextime now involves three to four million workers, most of them in white-collar jobs. Stanley Nollen (1979), professor of business economics at Georgetown University, analyzed findings from eight surveys covering 445 private and government organizations using flextime. He found that only 8 percent of the companies trying the innovation had dropped it. Reasons for "deflexing" included higher utility costs (for the longer workday) and opposition from supervisors. However, virtually no companies reported that the schedule slowed down production as had been feared.

On the contrary, Nollen found that 48 percent of the organizations reported productivity gains, averaging 12 percent. Most of the rest reported no change in productivity.

Few of the companies used control groups of non-flextime workers for comparison, which raises the question of whether a "Hawthorne effect" may have caused temporary gains in productivity through the novelty and attention surrounding the new program. However, when Nollen made his own calls to companies that had been using flextime for several years, they reported that the gains were holding up.

School administrators frequently have late afternoon and evening meetings. Perhaps a type of flextime might better accommodate their schedule.

Educational Solidarity

Martin Luther King said, "We must learn to live together as brothers or perish together as fools." Unfortunately, educators have ignored that advice and factioned themselves into various groups. There are now large, separate organizations for blue-collar, secretarial, teacher, support, and administrative staff members. Instead of combining forces to prevent further erosion of control over their own destiny, these groups have frequently polarized over territorial issues. By canceling one another's strengths, the groups have opened many opportunities for passage of restrictive state and federal legislation. The result has been debilitating initiative elections, general resistance and animosity by the public, less local control, and restriction of fiscal resources.

It would appear that the only possible solution to many educational ills is a concerted solidarity movement to bring about cooperation and combining of forces of all educational employees. Only then will issues like (1) reasonable local, state, and federal control, (2) a reasonable ratio of supervisors to staff, (3) realistic limitations regarding advisory councils, (4) adequate fiscal budgeting, and (5) control over student discipline be accomplished. If, for instance, it were determined that the funding level was so low that reasonable salaries, resources, and personnel could not be provided, then all schools and all employee groups might protest in concert.

Local Autonomy

Most school systems operate through a hierarchy of decision rendering. Often there is very little opportunity to solve problems that affect all employees. When control is limited by federal or state direction, morale and job satisfaction wane while burnout and distress grow. Local autonomy relieves frustration through mutual camaraderie and cooperation. Local school districts that are in control of their own budgets and curriculum can still maintain autonomous philosophy and policy.

The larger an organization becomes, the greater the strain placed on the total communication network. Many researchers recommend decentralization as a solution to the overall communication and decision-making problems in large organizations.

Delegation of Responsibility and Authority

School administrators and teachers should not try to pursue every task themselves. Many assignments, including most paper work, should be delegated to secretaries or assistants. Delegating a reasonable amount of work not only limits the possibility of work overload but conveys trust in others' capabilities. Giving others a chance to assume more responsibility strengthens them, provides training, variety, and an opportunity for recognition or eventual promotion. Thinking of oneself as the only person capable of doing the job is a faulty perception.

Delegation of work to staff should give them the opportunity to receive a project and take it to self-directed completion. This enables the individual to take full responsibility and allows the pride of accomplishment. A school administrator can foster this pride by assigning complete projects and allowing for individual autonomy. Including checkpoints along the way provides an opportunity for review and feedback. Pride and competence are engendered for both delegator and the recipient of the trust.

Other problems identified in Chapters V and VI—such as tenure, discipline, collective bargaining, students' rights movement, and so forth—are more complex and require the joint concerted efforts of legislators, community members, governing boards, teachers, employee organizations, administration, and students. This will be the case with other solution categories that follow.

ORGANIZATIONAL PRESCRIPTIONS FOR IMPROVED FEEDBACK/COMMUNICATION

Organizational Communication

The tone of organizational communication is obviously established at the top. If communication lines to and from top management are open and clear, an example is set for all inter- and intra-departmental communications. It is crucial for organizations to facilitate the sharing of information at all levels in order to keep people well informed and reinforce positive identification with the organization. A closed system of communication (except regarding items of a confidential nature) or one based on topdown hierarchies of communication is doomed to failure.

Communication should be both centralized and decentralized. Information about the organization as a whole should be shared from a central source. Information at each local level must also be provided, not only for the value of the information but also for recognition of employee achievement and feedback. An analysis of all levels of communication is an essential part of sound management. School managers at all levels must assume leadership for the communication process within their areas of responsibility.

A periodic review of organizational communication is helpful in determining areas of strength, as well as areas needing improvement. The following are general areas and suggested questions reflective of highly effective organizational communication.

Mutual Trust: Can staff members state their views and differences openly without fear of ridicule or retaliation? Can others disagree without intimidation or open attack?

Mutual Support: Do staff members provide unsolicited help to one another? Do colleagues rally around a team member who is in professional or personal need? Do staffs show open support for the policies and goals of the organization?

Mutual Communication: Do staff members express themselves freely to peers and supervisors without feeling guarded or cautious? Do others listen carefully and work toward understanding each other? Do individuals participate and accept responsibility to share necessary information?

Conflict Resolution: Do staff members perceive occasional conflict as necessary and desirable? Do team members work through appropriate solutions to conflict situations? Do staff members give advice or counsel when differences in values or perceptions conflict?

Use of Staff Resources: Are staff's abilities, knowledge, experience, and interests fully used within the school environment? Are individuals respected and valued for their differences?

Information flow is critical to an educational organization in order to assure and balance staff understanding and morale. An information flow chart should be developed after each recommendation or decision in order to identify what, who, how, and when information will be transmitted. Without a clear-cut two-way information flow, rumors will abound and insidiously undermine the best of organizational intention.

Public Awareness

Public awareness and support are a critical means of reducing distress. Researchers can compile data year after year, but if the public is not informed, the proposals and recommendations fall on deaf ears. Until the typical "person in the street" is educated, no political solutions will be found. Each local community can be strengthened by a school that fosters communication and involvement in school activities. People must be made aware; they must be provided with information if public education is to survive.

Staff Development

Staff cohesiveness can be developed by various feedback or communication approaches such as the following:

1. School staff members should be made to feel secure and should be able to express their ideas and emotions. Support from both peers and supervisors allows for expression of concerns and feelings without attack. The concept of the school supervisor meeting with individuals or groups and maintaining the ability to feel relaxed through two-way communication is extremely important.
2. Allowing for creativity through freedom for school employees to try new techniques is a supportive management practice. Encouraging and rewarding independent actions and providing means to assume such actions is often successful.
3. Providing ongoing feedback and guidance to fellow professionals reassures peers, supervisors, and subordinates that their existence is noticed and their contributions appreciated. Setting aside regular opportunities to provide informal as well as formal feedback is crucial. As mentioned earlier, everyone needs feedback and guidance in order to grow personally and professionally. It is important to let others know when they are doing a good job, as well as to provide constructive suggestions. It is sometimes helpful to keep a list of school staff members and mark each name when feedback is provided to that individual. This approach should assure feedback at least several times each week to every individual.
4. Participation by staff members in decision making should be directly and honestly encouraged. However, information should be requested only when it is to be used. Providing lip service to employee recommendations only backfires. As mentioned earlier, lack of participative decision making and limited autonomy are major causes of job distress. The involvement of staff insures total "ownership" by letting staff know their input was welcomed and determined the outcome of a situation.

Sally Reed ("Teacher Burnout," 1979b) reported that supervisors in Grand Forks, North Dakota have taken the offensive against teacher distress. They have designed a five-step program in which supervisors observe teachers to help them improve their teaching. Supervisors meet with teachers before and after each observation, giving feedback and suggestions for improvement of teacher-planned activities (p. 61).

Bridging the Gap Between Work and Home

Two and three generations ago, occupations usually involved the entire family. All family members played an important part not only in the work but in the play afterwards. Blacksmiths, carpenters, millers, and storekeepers all shared in the family enterprise of working, learning, and cooperating. There were few children who did not understand or were not able to explain the work of their parents. Today very few children can explain their parents' work. The gap between the work place and the home has reached monumental proportions.

School organizations should provide both awareness and on-the-job opportunities for families to visit, explore, and learn about their loved one's occupations. Almost all workers have pride in their jobs and want to share their accomplishments. Children need to learn about vocational preparedness. Work-social functions might be combined with job awareness activities so that families can participate in unity with their breadwinners. Associating work with family will further enhance a worker's pride and dignity. Allowing children to work alongside a parent for a few hours can sometimes complete a child's dream.

Community Interaction

An educator who has a close relationship with the school community has developed the necessary bond and support that makes his or her efforts worthwhile. Avoiding or withdrawing from the school community alienates those whose support is needed and destroys close, cooperative working relationships. The sense of community is too often missing in contemporary society. Schools should not only build internal support, but also provide external assistance to the entire community. This involvement and interaction gain momentum by clarifying a common purpose and sharing community objectives. A strong commitment of parents and staff working toward these commonalities for the good of the community and the school is necessary.

Communication and feedback are essential elements in the re-strengthening of community. Mortimer Feinberg ("Teacher Burnout," 1979b), aforementioned expert on burned out executives, suggests that the public attitude about schools must change. He stated:

Teachers, parents, and business community, must work towards raising the status of teachers in the professional field. The health of our education system depends on the effectiveness and mental attitudes of teachers. We'll have fewer burned out teachers when they begin to feel they have an importance in the future of the nation. (p. 62)

Fear of Violence

Many school employees face a serious problem today—the possibility of violence. The fear of violence is quite real for school personnel (see discussion in Chapter VI). Schools must be prepared to deal with both internal and external turbulence. Plans should be available both to prevent and to deal with violent crises. The coordination of administrators, teachers, psychologists/counselors, parents, and community workers to keep the schools safe is important, and planning efforts should not be ignored. If staff members are prepared and know what to do under these circumstances, they will feel safer and unnecessary stress can be prevented.

ORGANIZATIONAL PRESCRIPTIONS FOR WORK OVERLOAD

Reduced Supervisory Ratios

Perhaps the most blatant and obvious cause of stress in education is the ratio of supervisors to staff. Many researchers have noted that as the number of people for whom a given individual is responsible increases, greater cognitive, sensory, and emotional overload results. Careful analysis of work responsibilities, particularly the number of people a manager directly supervises, should be conducted at least once a year.

Take a Break, Sabbatical, Leave of Absence, "Shared Contract"

Everyone needs an occasional short break from a difficult job. A sabbatical, leave of absence, or shared contract can provide breathing time to reorganize priorities. An opportunity to establish new life and work goals is often necessary, especially when energy has been drained through the demands of excellent performance. A structured break is a powerful tool to accomplish personal and professional growth. Coming back to work refreshed, with renewed vigor and a relaxed attitude, helps both the individual and the organization.

The sabbatical leave has been a traditional safeguard against burnout. Likewise, a leave of absence or a shared contract is an excellent way to keep professionally active without burning out. Obviously these alternative work plans need not always be a year's duration, but might be creatively designed for a partial year or semester. Truch (1980) suggests that a sabbatical be granted every seven or eight years. It could be financed by a nominal monthly deduction for that purpose.

In Palo Alto, California, teachers are able to take a year off to pursue a special project under a program called Project Renew. In other areas of the country, school boards and administrators are helping employees start exchange programs with educators in other areas. Grants and fellowships also offer similar breaks.

The shared contract is another increasingly popular form of partial leave. Rather than leaving the profession entirely, many good teachers are working part-time by sharing a position and thereby using the greatest professional strengths of each.

Cutting Back on Projects

The proliferation of new educational projects in the past ten years is astounding. Some administrators feel they and their staffs can no longer continue to add new programs. Instead they are beginning to look for ways to peel off some. Adding one constraint after another without taking any away causes classic work overload. With the ever-increasing load of paper work, it would be wise for school boards and administrators to review the various "laundry lists" with the intention of eliminating rather than adding projects. Escalating public and legislative demands create an urgent need for top management to help teachers, principals, and support staff members relieve pressure by cutting unnecessary tasks and consolidating others. The satisfaction of working with children and helping them grow will be enhanced if more undivided attention can be given to the youngsters rather than to bureaucratic details.

Early or Partial Retirement

Many school districts have elected to help teachers and administrators plan for early retirement. School employees who are 55 or older can elect to work 20–50 days each year at a task mutually acceptable to both the individual and the district. These extra days' pay plus retirement provide enough income to make early retirement desirable. Not only are costs to the district cut, but educators have a chance to phase out with dignity and self-respect.

Support for a Stress Management Program

According to Morrison (1977), administrators who participate in stress-management seminars and establish a self-management plan have reaped highly positive results. More importantly, their supervisors were surprised to find that such personal expansion did not detract from but rather contributed to work effectiveness. Instead of becoming self-indulgent, supervisors reported more task-oriented behaviors and more sensitivity to other's needs. School officials should encourage individual, as well as organizational, stress management programs.

Variety of Tasks

Participation in a range of activities can be more stress-releasing than spending each day with a highly limited focus. Participating in a range of activities will provide variety within an organization. A balance of paper work, direct contact with people, development of new or refined programs, participation in committees, or shared decision making offers variety and wards off the effects of monotony or burnout. An individual's choice of activities can dramatically assist in avoiding distress.

Additional Assistance

Teachers regularly take attendance, count noses for lunch, inventory books, correct papers, and record information. Some teachers hire older students to assist in correcting papers and doing routine clerical work. Some secondary schools provide teacher assistants as part of a work-study program for students. Some principals have established a rotating system of administrative coverage and assistance that shares this responsibility with willing teachers. Some schools have organized internal teams to assist in accomplishing administrative functions such as supervision, accountability, guidance, and informal evaluation/ feedback to fellow teachers. Any creative means of low-cost assistance is helpful in warding off work overload, as well as in providing variety and training for others.

ORGANIZATIONAL PRESCRIPTIONS FOR CONTACT OVERLOAD

Review of Caseload

Constant contact with difficult and needy people, like contact sports, can be dangerous to the health of employees. Periodic review of caseloads (especially for school counselors, psychologists, social workers, and vice-principals) is helpful in determining the need for job re-engineering. When a job involves almost continual contact with needy or difficult individuals (e.g., students, parents, or even colleagues), consideration should be given to other non-contact tasks. Providing for a certain amount of paper work or more creative interludes will help bring variety and relief.

Additional Training for High Contact

Maslach (1976) found clear research evidence that individuals who have close contact with people need more training and preparation than others not working in close relationships to people. Unfortunately, educational training institutions provide only minimal course work related to dealing with difficult or needy individuals. In addition, few educators have had experience dealing with the variety of difficult personalities or the range of intense emotions found in a typical school community. Schools are special in that the unique focus of work is children. Children represent, in many ways, the emotional extensions and egos of parents. A parent may become upset over a faulty product purchased from a store, but seldom does the emotion ever approach the wrath generated by a real or imagined injustice to his or her child. Training to prepare educators more effectively for intensive contact with needy or difficult people is of utmost necessity.

ORGANIZATIONAL PRESCRIPTIONS FOR JOB CONFLICT/AMBIGUITY

Expectations/Role Conflict

School organizations should clearly establish their expectations of employees. Both long-range (three to five years) as well as short-range goals (three to ten months) need clarification. Delineation of job functions, amount of time available, staffing patterns, and schedules must be clearly and specifically worked out. School boards, for example, should clearly establish their immediate objectives and long-range goals before the beginning of each school year. This clarity will assist school administrators in developing specific management objectives that can be measured by year end. If, in the interim of accomplishing these educational goals, new programs or goals creating job conflict are established, some effort must be made to remove or limit the earlier job requirements. This acknowledgment provides individuals with recognition that their needs have been taken into consideration at the time of newly established courses of action. The school staff and organization can function optimally only if there is a trusting, mutually caring environment.

Mutual Cooperation

It has been stated, "A house divided against itself cannot stand." As school districts grow in size, departments or related organizations often become insulated from each other. In order to achieve maximum effectiveness, all subsections and related organizations must be enlisted in a common effort. Institutions of higher education, state departments of education, legislators, local school districts, professional organizations, and industrial/business enterprises must work together. Representatives of each should select one or two high priorities that can be mutually solved by close cooperation.

Such cooperation may assist state legislators and departments of education in working together rather than independent of one another. Working together may assist in a return to completing tasks with a sensible simplicity rather than setting up complex, overlapping entities. Most important, however, might be the replacement of mutual complaint with mutual support. Legislators and educators need to support each other if there is to be success in improving education and service to the community.

Job Re-engineering

Job re-engineering includes job task analysis and redesign. By periodically redefining job objectives, conditions, and content, the school organization can optimize both productivity and employee satisfaction. This process simply enriches the educator's job by making periodic revisions and improvements. For example, spelling may be determined as a high priority subject area needing teacher restructuring. Specific methods and materials might be developed by a local school or district with input, ownership, and support from all involved.

Job objectives and conditions should take into account the needs of not only the organization but the school employee. Likewise, educational materials (textbooks, electronic aids, etc.), as the tools of the employee, need to be reviewed if productivity is to be enhanced. By clearly defining objectives with the assistance of the employee, by analyzing job conditions and reviewing the necessary materials, the focus is placed upon the employee as well as the organization (something learned from the Hawthorne studies). Quick and Quick (1979) strongly support job redesign as a means to increase new opportunities for achievement, responsibility, and recognition. They report that both productivity and morale increase after such re-engineering. It is also advisable to test each new job redesign and reevaluate its effectiveness over an extended period.

Organizational Restructuring

When a job has been identified as providing little autonomy, minimal opportunity for participation, and little job satisfaction, a partial organizational restructuring is necessary. School organizations committed to distress abatement should build in periodic reviews of various educational job classifications that need organizational restructuring. For example, a review of the ratio of supervisors to the number of personnel they evaluate might be called for. It could be determined that a more efficient grouping would be work units of eight. Each unit would be chaired by a rotating or assigned person who received extra pay and recognition for coordination and supervision. Another example of an area that might need reorganizing would be the "division of labor" in curriculum areas.

Such restructuring is also necessary if high technology, legal, or social changes have occurred at a rapid rate (e.g., use of computers and video tape for instruction or evaluation). Ongoing training and job renewal activities are necessary if organizational restructuring is to be successful. Continual clarification of roles and interpersonal relationships can be accomplished by ongoing communication and "feedback loops." As with stress reduction, restructuring can only be accomplished if there is first a perception of the need for readjustment.

Rotation

As mentioned earlier, "People are like tires, they need to be rotated periodically!" At Rockford Elementary School in Rockford, Minnesota, teachers switch grades periodically. This practice breaks up routines and provides new challenges.

Organizations expect that individuals will work cooperatively and harmoniously together. This is enhanced by directly experiencing and empathizing with the importance of each worker's role. When a teacher complains about a custodian or principal, it is often because the complainer has had little experience with those jobs. The fear of new situations can be lessened by many role experiences at school.

In a democratic nation that prides itself on equality, it is important that individuals become humble enough to accept and understand the toil of their brethren. Faculty members should have an opportunity (even though it might be short) to be a teacher, administrator, psychologist, custodian, secretary, aide, and special educator. Awareness and understanding of others' roles only become real when these roles are role-played rather than merely discussed. If teenagers can take on the function of a city mayor, city manager, treasurer, and so forth, educators can participate in role rotation. Likewise, students in vocational education programs can and should assume the role of teachers, administrators, custodians, or cooks.

ORGANIZATIONAL PRESCRIPTIONS REGARDING INDIVIDUAL FACTORS

Hiring

If optimal educational results are desired, the fit between job description and individual employee should be as close as possible. Ideally, once the job description has been clearly defined, a search should be conducted for the best available person. When a job is matched with an appropriate person and the seven major occupational stressors are controlled, other problems can be minimized. As jobs and situations change, school administrators should continually intervene and promote reevaluation of an individual's strengths and weaknesses. This facilitation provides growth for new and related jobs as they become available.

Tolerance of Imperfection

Since distress is an individual perception, it is often rooted in perceived imperfection. Many organizations and their managers experience an unnecessary amount of distress because they fail to accept imperfection in themselves, others, or the work environment. Under critical scrutiny, it might seem that everything is imperfect. Individuals who accept imperfection or weakness can minimize the effects of stress. Focusing upon how much improvement is made rather than upon how far there is yet to go provides optimism. The process of converting negative energy ("it's half empty") into positive energy ("it's half full") is based upon revised perceptions and attitudes.

Professional or Personal Development

For many years it was an organizational myth that the major function of a company was to train individuals to be better employees by providing training in strictly work-related areas. Some 50 years ago, beginning with the Hawthorne studies, it was found that attention paid to individual employees provided a new frame of reference—namely self-motivated personal development. Since that time, many organizations have found that providing personal development opportunities to staff pays huge dividends. Giving employees a chance to attend classes and learn better skills in communications or management helps them not only to become better workers, but also to become better people. In one study of 14 major industries (Cedoline, 1980), it was found that the average manager undertook 40–60 hours of training per year. Much of this training related to personal, as well as professional, development. If the organization takes responsibility for each employee's personal and professional growth, it strengthens both the organization and the society within which it functions.

Matching Organizational Needs with Personal Goals

In order to successfully match organizational needs with personal goals, the following conditions should be considered.

1. School assignments should be reasonably demanding and offer variety.
2. The position should provide for the need to learn on the job and to continue to learn.
3. The educational setting should provide some areas of decision making that an individual can call his or her own.
4. The work environment should provide some degree of social support, recognition, and feedback.
5. The educator's job should provide a relationship between work and outside activities.
6. The school-related job should help create a desirable future for both the individual and for society as a whole.

Career Planning/Pathing

Each professional employee deserves a periodic (at least once every three years) opportunity to review individual and professional strengths. At this time it should be determined what might be projected for the next three years. Opportunities for transfer, promotion, or reassignment should be explored. Emphasis on personal and professional growth should be directed toward desired career changes. Voluntary and planned change is often rewarding, but difficult; involuntary and unplanned change is frequently destructive and contributes to failure. If change is planned and realistically projected (allowing for adequate preparation), success will often be achieved. Change can be in the form of emphasizing special skills, developing new competencies, making lateral or promotional moves, or simply changing the working environment.

ORGANIZATIONAL PRESCRIPTIONS
FOR TRAINING DEFICITS

Advocates/Mentors

The Orleans Parish school system in New Orleans employs eight teacher advocates as an important part of its staff-development program. New teachers can call upon the advocates confidentially for help with curriculum and discipline problems. Advocates also work with teacher selection committees and provide inservice activities. The program has paid large dividends. There have been significantly fewer resignations among new teachers since its inception.

In Palo Alto a project called Personal Help Center provides short-term confidential consultations with teachers. In some cases this program has saved teachers' careers, as well as encouraged better teaching performance.

The Chicago Teachers Union provides a self-help center and health program for teachers under distress. A teacher crisis center in New York is currently being prepared. "Born-again teachers" have resulted from such offerings as "Revival," provided by a teacher center in Connecticut.

Advocates for teachers or administrators should be selected from a pool of seasoned, highly competent professionals. These skilled educators might temporarily delegate their regular jobs to others (providing themselves variety and time out) in order to assist peers in need, particularly new or less effective employees.

Specialized Training

Before an industrial worker is entrusted to command machinery or to perform certain skilled labor, a license or certificate of competence is often required. In contrast, management of people requires little or no evidence of competence in the important areas of psychology, sociology, or occupational health. An analogy is often made that equates parents and managers. You need a license to drive, but need demonstrate almost no required competence to be a parent or manager. A logical solution might be to provide prospective managers a minimum of compulsory, specialized education. Such specialized education is desperately needed to prepare managers for making responsible decisions and for assisting their employees in monitoring and evaluating healthful progress. In addition, ongoing specialized training is necessary for both renewal and survival within ever-changing educational functions.

Team Building/Quality Control Groups

Certain industrial firms, particularly successful Japanese companies, have found great benefit from a concept developed by the Union of Japanese Scientists and Engineers called "QC Groups." This team-building technique allows a facilitator—usually a trained outsider—to meet with representatives within a department. The objectives are to: identify departmental needs; develop successful means of problem solving; increase internal communication; resolve work-related problems; enhance morale and good feelings for the organization; and increase productivity. Managers increase their understanding of the human needs within their departments ("content"), as well as participate in the group's collaborative change ("process").

The QC concept validates the original Hawthorne studies, which found that the more attention is paid to employees, the more sustained productivity results. In addition, it provides both training and an opportunity to participate in problem solving, which prevent two major sources of distress.

Ongoing Training

Organizations need to recognize that training and treatment are complementary. Training replenishes individuals, not only with new knowledge, but also with sources of creative energy which often have been depleted.

Research strongly suggests that professionals need continued specialized training for working closely with people. When faced with repeated, intense, emotional interactions with people, workers need constant retraining to avoid total detachment or conflict.

In addition, educators need to develop new skills, including new methods to accomplish old tasks. The following areas have been determined by a California Task Force to be at least a starting point for ongoing training (Mangers, 1978).

1. Stress Management
2. Shared Decision Making
3. Time Management
4. Leadership Activities in Today's World
5. Needs' Assessment
6. Participative Management/Decentralized Decision Making/ Problem Solving
7. Improving Community Support/Public Relations
8. Advisory Committees
9. Collective Bargaining/Grievance Procedures
10. Organizational Development and Change
11. Communication Skills
12. Program Review and Evaluation
13. Various Discipline Procedures
14. Parent Education
15. Inservice Opportunities
16. Utilization of Available Resources
17. Politics of Management
18. General Management in Today's Schools (Writing, Speaking, Planning, Delegating)

The improvement of training through inservice workshops can be accomplished by establishing rotating cadres of administrators and teachers assigned to work on current and anticipated needs.

Loaned Educators

Many school systems exist in geographic proximity. Each may employ highly skilled administrators, teachers, counselors, and other employees with various special talents. It is common for boards of education to need the temporary services of one or more of these specialists from another district. These talented individuals can: start a new program; "debug" a beginning or ongoing program; provide advice or counsel on needed techniques in identified areas; train a cadre of local staff; solve problems; model a new administrative skill or teaching behavior; spark innovation and creativity; or provide "new blood" or change to an otherwise good system gone stale.

Bringing in an educator on a short-term loan basis avoids a permanent loss of valuable talent to one school organization, while benefiting another system. This concept is similar to a company's loan of key employees to other firms or to a government agency for a special purpose. This process can be made reciprocal by a temporary trade of needed educators between school systems. The benefits are not only to the organization; they add to an individual's personal and professional growth.

Prior Understanding of Possible Distressful Conditions

The preventative approach of providing information to a new educator about possible occupational distress is helpful in decreasing its effects. This can be accomplished by an experienced staff member counseling a new staff member. Educators also need an opportunity to review highly distressful situations with colleagues to discover and share other methods of coping. Understanding will increase the worker's resistance to distress. Distressed school employees can be assisted by understanding and through peer support, which moderates negative effects. The old adage "an ounce of prevention is worth a pound of cure" is certainly appropriate to occupational distress.

SUMMARY

Simply stated, good personnel management requires a match between the individual and the organization. This can be accomplished by means of careful personnel selection or through individualized training and preparation. In the past ten years, the question of the quality of work life has been gaining the attention of top management. The National Center for Productivity and Quality of Working Life in Houston, Texas, has focused upon efforts to improve the work place by making it more human. Programs of stress reduction have been initiated by some large corporations. In order to sustain these new efforts, it will be necessary to educate and train employees to deal effectively with stress. Where appropriate, employers must begin to re-engineer the work environment by identifying the major causes of stress and then applying workable solutions. When organizations place the worker at the same level of priority as the profit that flows from their product or services, they will then have made an optimal match between the individual and the organization's objectives.

Organizational objectives focus upon individual productivity and competency. In order to accomplish these objectives, optimal motivating stress and reasonable compensation, as well as respect for the welfare, values, and needs of the employee, are necessary. An optimal match between person and organization must:

- Provide autonomy and decision-making opportunities that will offer control over one's own destiny;
- Maintain excellent two-way communication with the employee and provide immediate feedback;
- Regulate quantitative and qualitative work load;
- Be cognizant of and make necessary adjustments for contact overload;
- Clarify job roles to prevent conflict and ambiguity;
- Provide adequate training in technical, interpersonal, and other work-related areas;
- Provide opportunities for individuals to use their strengths and skills fully.

CHAPTER X

Organizational Development
and
Inservice Training

ORGANIZATIONAL DEVELOPMENT

Organizational development has been widely practiced in industry during the past two decades. The concept has only recently begun to receive recognition and attention within school systems. In fact, organizational change within education has occurred mainly through accident or pragmatic analysis of what did or did not work. Organizational development is a participatory data-based process for improving working relationships, programs, student learning, and climate when utilized within a school organization (Martin, Roark, & Tonso, 1978).

The purpose of organizational development is to promote effectiveness within all levels of an organization. This is accomplished by maximizing productivity and personal satisfaction via individual and organizational change and mutual growth. Specific areas of focus that achieve this improved quality of work life are:

- Development of clear and open communication at all levels by establishment of new communication skills.
- Establishment of mutual trust through increased understanding and better communication.
- Determination that human relations development and systematic goal setting are major goals of all organizations.
- Involvement of more individuals in decision making and encouragement of information and nonjudgmental identification of problems.

- Creation of an open problem-solving climate of mutual cooperation and collaboration.
- Development of group effectiveness through group tasks.
- Establishment of procedures that allow conflict to emerge and comfortably encourage resolution.
- Commitment to a total system effort.

The above areas can be successfully accomplished only if involvement, commitment, planning, and funding are supported by the entire work force—particularly top level managers. Maximum progress can be achieved by the use of an outside consultant to assist in the organizational development process.

In school systems as well as in all organizations, problems occur when informal (unwritten or personal) values come into conflict with formal goals. Such conflicts severely disrupt school effectiveness. Organizational development effectively works toward reducing the size, number, and effect of conflicts. The process is begun by systematically assessing the situation at all levels (e.g., staff, community, students). When needs are identified, then goals are established which are to be implemented through cooperative action.

Successful implementation within the organizational development concept is dependent upon agreed-upon procedures and activities. Individuals need to be clear about what they are doing, how they are doing it, and their feelings about the procedures. For example, if assertive discipline has been adopted by a school staff as a compatible goal, it is important to determine how consistently it is being carried out by teachers. Similarly it must be determined how effective the system is in decreasing disruptive behavior and how much staff support has been generated by the new system. In public education the organizational development process can be complicated because the community may not have clearly decided upon compatible goals (e.g., consensus about discipline policy).

Obviously, before successful assertive discipline goals and implementation are determined, valid information must be collected to permit accurate definition of the problem. This might include number of discipline referrals, suspensions, amount of staff time devoted to discipline, etc. The ultimate purpose of organizational development is to insure involvement of staff in decision making and support of mutually determined goals and procedures.

Objectives

According to Roark and Davis (1980) there are four primary objectives of organizational development. These are:

1. To provide a fit between the organization's goals and procedures, e.g., teaching writing skills by lecturing is a poor fit.
2. To relieve the tension between individual autonomy and organizational constraints. This tension is inevitable since individuals strive for autonomy while the organization strives for control. If there is too much constraint, individual creativity and intelligence are stifled, e.g., teachers cried "foul" when one school district put in time clocks.
3. To provide a fit between the task and process, e.g., when the auditorium is available, showing a film to 120 students instead of only 20 students.
4. To balance the quality of data with informed choices and adequate planning, e.g., the fairly common practice of arbitrarily rotating principals among schools without a plan or without involvement of principals in the decision.

In addition to these four primary objectives, organizational development usually addresses other specific and overlapping issues. These include: leadership, decision making, problem solving, conflict management, communication, and planning. Again the goal of organizational development is to improve the quality of life in the organization. A main function is to provide team building which builds interpersonal relationships by improved cooperation, communication, and conflict management.

Organizational Development Sequence

The sequence of organizational development intervention includes: entry, diagnosis, planning, implementation, assessment, and disengagement.

Entry is achieved by gaining acceptance, credibility, and trust. A valid two-way sharing of information, an understanding of organizational development, and an analysis of the initial level and type of communication are crucial. As trust and credibility grow, a working contract must be accomplished before successful entry is achieved. The contract contains the general requirements and enough specific (e.g., time commitments) to the intervention so that all parties understand in advance and that an initial commitment is made.

Diagnosis involves the collection of data as soon as possible. It can be obtained through casual conversations, questionnaires, interviews, review of records, etc. Diagnosis helps to define conditions, feelings, and desires. As many individuals as possible should be solicited to assist in data collection.

Planning is essential because the subsequent steps need to be developed as well as accepted so that intervention can be supported and maintained.

Implementation is not merely employment of the plan but a carefully planned procedure that allows for ongoing feedback, inservice education, checkpoints, course corrections, meetings, and resolution of new problems related to the intervention.

Assessment both determines the impact of the intervention and provides an analysis of the current state of the organization. The state of the organization needs to be measured to determine the effects of organizational development intervention.

Disengagement simply concludes the organizational development intervention by withdrawal.

Available Resources

Currently there are:

- 100,000 university and college professors for 2 million classroom teachers (or about one per 20 teachers).
- 100,000 principals and vice principals in the 17,000 school districts (or again another one per 20 teachers).
- 50,000 non-supervisory instructional personnel (e.g., media communications and/or reading instructors, mental health specialists).
- In addition, teachers are themselves the most valuable resource for each other. Service as mentor and coach is vital to their continued development.

If only 10 percent of their time was devoted to inservice education, the effect upon staff would be incalculable.

INSERVICE TRAINING

From the years 1940 to 1970, the numbers involved in American education grew at an incredible rate. The teaching force alone increased from one million to over two million. Schools of education bulged and production of teachers exceeded the size of the demand; one-third of the education candidates never sought employment and another third left the profession within three years. Consequently, teacher preparation became brief, chaotic, and frequently inadequate (Joyce, Yarger, & Howey, 1977).

With increased births and population, school districts were opening schools at a rapid rate. Often teachers and counselors with little administrative experience were promoted to principalships. Meanwhile, schools were staffed with relatively young and inexperienced teachers. At the same time came calls for higher quality prompted by the Soviet launching of Sputnik and the publication of Rudolf Flesch's book *Why Johnny Can't Read* (1966).

By 1970 the pace slowed substantially due to decreased school enrollments. An aroused public began to see the schools as not only less effective but too costly. Teachers in the meantime had begun to organize and unionize over economic and work condition issues. Both educators and the public became angry about the conditions of our schools. Considerable concern was voiced regarding the serious shortcomings of professional growth and development. Substantial research by local, state, and federal agencies was conducted and yielded a great deal about teaching and schooling (Joyce & Morine, 1977). What was found was that substantial continuous staff development was essential for the improvement, renewal, and survival of public education. If free public education is to survive as a vital function of American society, it will be necessary to rebuild the school into a life-long learning laboratory for both children and teachers. The most important focus suggested by the research was on learning how to learn.

In an age of rapid change, even the best conceivable preservice education cannot sustain an educator for more than four to six years. One author observed that immediately upon graduation from a training institution, educators embark upon a journey of obsolescence (Rubin, 1975, pp. 31–38).

In industry, as well as in bureaucracies such as the military or professions such as medicine, it is recognized that extensive ongoing training is necessary. All recognize that the updating of skills and knowledge needs to be carefully planned, ordered, monitored, and maintained. In medicine, medical boards and centers offer a variety of seminars and workshops for all health professionals. Major industrial corporations have elaborate training centers and expend substantial amounts of money to train personnel.

Although educators recognize a need for continuous training, staff development efforts are frequently ineffective, poorly conceived, and inadequately financed. Rubin suggests that better inservice definition and planning are needed. Inservice programs should be based upon practical factors as well as research findings.

Wood, Thompson, and Russell (1981) reported that the design of an inservice plan is shaped by a number of assumptions supported by research data:

1. All personnel in schools, to stay current and effective, need and should be involved in inservice training throughout their careers.
2. Significant improvement in educational practice takes considerable time and is the result of systematic, long-range staff development (e.g., short-term workshops are only part of a major inservice plan).
3. Inservice education should have an impact on the quality of the school program and focus on helping staff improve their abilities to perform their professional responsibilities (Edelfelt, 1977).
4. Adult learners are motivated to risk learning new behaviors when they believe they have control over the learning situation and are free from threat of failure (Withall & Wood, 1979).
5. Educators vary widely in their professional competencies, readiness, and approaches to learning, i.e., inservice programs need to accommodate individual differences.
6. Professional growth requires personal and group commitment to new performance, i.e., changes in behavior are the result of willingness to change.
7. Organizational health (including factors such as social climate, trust, open communication and peer support for change) influences the success of inservice programs.
8. The school is the primary unit of change, not the district or the individual, i.e., the individual teacher is too isolated and too small a unit to ensure sustained change.
9. School districts have the primary responsibility for providing the resources and training necessary for a school staff to implement new programs and improve instruction.
10. The school principal is the gatekeeper for adoption and continued use of new practices and programs in a school, i.e., commitment, participation, encouragement, implementation, monitoring, and maintenance.

Wood, Thompson, and Russell view the optimal inservice program as having five distinct but related stages. These stages include Readiness, Planning, Training, Implementation, and Maintenance.

Readiness

Readiness is often the most forgotten stage of staff development. At this initial level school climate and support are developed. During the readiness phase, staffs determine problems, possible solutions, and procedures to be used. Support is generated by open communication, allowing time, participation, commitment to change, and trust in leadership. The results of readiness include inservice goals, general practices selected to achieve goals, and a broad four-to-five year plan to implement these long-term goals.

Planning

Joyce and Peck (1977) indicated that teachers, administrators, and university instructors feel the major defect in an inservice training program often has been poor organization and planning. Adequate planning requires the development of a detailed long-range plan which is refined into specific inservice objectives. It is based upon needs assessment, activities needed, and procurement of resources. It is the who, what, where, and when of inservice training. Leadership during planning should be shared between individual staff members and administrators. It is important that an adequate budget to support the long-range inservice program be available and protected for the duration.

Training

During this stage the inservice plan is carried out. The content, skills, and attitudes needed to implement changes in professional behavior are learned during training. Orientation activities provide participants with a clear understanding of specific objectives, sequence of activities, expectations, options, relevance to school needs, and follow up on a day-to-day basis. "Warm up" activities are often provided to develop a climate of cooperation.

At this stage learning teams or groups are established and baseline or entry level skills of participants are charted for later comparison. Also, it is important to allow participants some selection of activities and materials. Participants should also devise a tentative plan for implementing what has been learned into their daily activities and for practicing their new behaviors and skills. School principals remain key and pivotal people in school improvement and change.

Teachers or principals who develop expertise and are approved as skilled trainers can become inservice leaders for a school district. They can receive released time, leadership stipends, and special recognition to compensate them for their skill and time providing inservice.

Implementation

Actual on-the-job implementation of newly learned skills should begin as soon as possible. When participants leave a workshop, a written plan for implementing their learning should accompany them. Obviously, a substantial amount of assistance is needed when educators first attempt to use the new skill on a regular basis. A cadre of school staff should be on call to assist in problem solving, sharing, and supporting. Regular meetings should provide an opportunity for feedback and problem resolution. Administrative support and recognition as well as budgeting for essential resources is important throughout implementation. Recognition can be provided by newspaper or school newsletter releases, additional travel, opportunity to become an inservice leader for others, or released time to work out problems.

Maintenance

Any new behavior cannot be considered permanent even when it has initially become part of an ongoing school activity. Maintenance is the establishment of a continuous process for monitoring to insure that the new behaviors are practiced and that established goals are met. Monitoring can be provided by checklists, observation, video or audio recording interviews, and ongoing surveys. A coordinating committee in each school can also provide ongoing maintenance.

Wood, Thompson, and Russell (1981) summarized the critical characteristics of staff development:

- Inservice education should be conducted in a supportive climate of trust, peer support, open communication, and staff commitment to a set of clearly understood norms for functioning in an institution (clear roles, program definition, instruction procedures, goals).
- Inservice education goals should be based upon a common set of expectations held by the participants that are essential to performing their professional roles in their institution.
- Successful inservice education requires support from administration and school boards including time, personnel, training materials, and funds to enable the training necessary to implement educational programs.
- Decisions concerning the objectives, experiences, and assessment of inservice education should be cooperatively developed by those involved in and affected by the training program.
- Inservice education should be based upon assessed needs of participants. A need is defined as a gap between the expected professional performance and actual performance in the work setting.
- Inservice education should model the instructional behaviors desired of participants.
- Inservice education programs should be demanding and set high but reasonable standards of performance for participants.

- Inservice education programs should have three major components: (1) attitude, (2) pedagogical skills, and (3) substantive knowledge.
- Inservice education should prepare educators to implement research findings and develop the best practices related to carrying out their job responsibilities.
- Inservice education should be decentralized; focus on actual school problems, goals, needs, and plans; and be conducted, whenever feasible, in the school setting.
- Inservice education should emphasize use of rewards (such as opportunity, increased autonomy, participation in decision making, increased competence, success, and advancement) which have been shown to promote high commitment and performance.
- Inservice education should be based upon clear, well understood, specific goals and objectives that are congruent with institutional and personal goals.
- Inservice education should provide options for participants that will accommodate individual professional needs and learning styles (timing, sequence, pace, interests, goals, delivery systems).
- Inservice education should be experientially based with opportunities to select, adapt, and try out new professional behaviors in real and simulated work settings.
- Central office personnel and school administrators should support inservice education through their participation in training activities with their peers and subordinates.
- Inservice education programs should provide for follow-up and "on call" assistance to educators as they use their new skills and understandings in the work setting after they have been trained.
- Leadership in inservice education programs should be situational and emphasize authority by competence and expertise rather than by position.
- Evaluation of inservice education should be both formative and summative and should examine the immediate effect on participants, extent of transfer to the work setting, and the effect on achieving institutional goals.

CHAPTER XI

Profiles of Success

Until a few years ago, doctors and laymen traditionally assumed that top executives are the most prone to stress. Recent studies show, however, that top executives (those who have "made it") seem to thrive on distress, and have a better chance of living longer lives than middle managers or junior executives. A 16-year study conducted by Metropolitan Life Insurance Company of New York of those occupying the top three positions in *Fortune* magazine's top 500 corporations showed them to have a mortality rate of only 63 percent of the general white male population (West, 1978).

J. P. McCann, medical board chairman of an organization that administers physical examinations to executives of more than 1500 companies, says that top executives are among the healthiest people in America. Instead, he sees many more signs of distress among middle managers (West, 1978).

A survey of four levels of school administration revealed that job satisfaction correlated with one's position in the hierarchy (Brown, 1976). Only two levels of satisfaction were distinguished. Principal and central office directors enjoyed their work least—assistant superintendents and superintendents enjoyed their work most.

Los Angeles Business and Economics published an excellent article, "How Chief Executives Handle Stress" (West, 1978). Nationally known executives of large corporations who have learned successful coping strategies were interviewed. Some of the responses* included:

Barron Hilton, president, Hilton Hotels Corporation:

---

* Reprinted by permission of Nedra West, Editor, *Los Angeles Business and Economics,* © 1978.

In my judgment, the degree of stress that an executive experiences, in the conduct of his or her responsibilities, is directly related to the preparation of confidence with which the individual approaches each new business challenge.

I have long subscribed to the philosophy that worry solves nothing. As a result, I approach each business opportunity with the interest and excitement of a new challenge. While the pace and intensity of my efforts may cause my adrenaline to flow faster, I look upon such an experience as one of enjoyment rather than one of stress.

In my own case, I think the closest I come to answering the question of how I handle stress lies in the importance I attach to periods of relaxation and total escape from what I look upon as the pace of business. I find that relaxation and total escape in the peace and quiet of a weekend of soaring in my sailplane, or in my hobbies of golf, hunting and nature photography. In turn, those opportunities for total relaxation recharge my energies and leave me eager to return to the challenge of business.

Donn B. Tatum, chairman of the board, Walt Disney Productions:

Coping with strain and stress is primarily a matter of mental pacing and discipline, much the same as anything else. The discipline consists of learning to expect it, training one's self to recognize it when it appears, and, the hardest part, forcing one's self to turn it off and direct one's thoughts to something else so as to provide a balance.

Harry J. Volk, chairman, Union Bank:

One handles tension best, I believe, by putting problems in their perspective with respect to the total success of a business and with respect to all those things which ultimately bring happiness and contentment in personal living. One must remember that problems eventually are solved and difficult situations are handled and corrected.

Some problems which result in tensions exist only for a short time; others continue for longer periods. The chief executive has to be aware of the fact that problems will ever be arising. He can best cope with the resulting tension and stress if he has continuing appreciation of the fact that problems will arise and that he can find solutions.

In coping with stress, he must maintain his health by dismissing problems from his mind when he is away from the office. He must eat and drink intelligently, exercise reasonably, engage in activities in which he finds enjoyment, and use moderation in everything he does.

A competent, intelligent, emotionally stable chief executive finds the stress from a continuing stream of problems just as manageable as an emotionally stable housewife and mother would find handling stress arising from managing a family.

J. R. Fluor, chairman, Fluor Corporation:

I have developed the capability of making decisions as required with the ability to go on to others things.

I am blessed with the body chemistry that allows me to go to sleep easily and awaken refreshed, whether on an airplane, at home, or a short rest during the noon hour.

I have the temperament that permits me to work through others in accomplishing a tremendous amount of work in a relaxed atmosphere.

I have an exercise program which I do both morning and evening.

I have hobbies and interests outside my business life. Golf is particularly relaxing even though I do not play even once a week on the average due to a heavy business travel schedule.

Verne H. Winchell, chairman and president, Denny's, Inc.:

I had to stop and think, just how do I handle stress? Of course, it is something that has grown over the years. It isn't something that happened overnight—anyway not to me. Adding responsibilities in small increments is much healthier than taking on too much too fast.

I find that being involved in many activities gives me relief from the others. I derive a great deal of pleasure, for instance, from the thoroughbred horse breeding business. It is very different from my day-to-day business, so I find it relaxing. I also find great relaxation and challenge in playing the organ and piano. But I guess the main thing is I enjoy going from one activity to another.

At this point in my life, being so involved in so many different areas, I rely on responsible associates to handle the day-to-day details, which allows me to work on the planning level which I enjoy. Delegating as much as possible allows me to be involved, but not burdened. I think another reason I am able to accomplish a great deal with relatively little stress is I am very interested in what I am doing, and being successful doing it helps make it very enjoyable.

R. Parker Sullivan, president, General Telephone Company of California:

Long ago I made up my mind that I would not allow tension and stress to create problems for my mental, physical, or emotional well-being. In the first place, stress and tension can only hinder a person's ability to think and make decisions. Secondly, I believe tension and stress are underlying causes for other more serious problems.

Following some time of experimentation I arrived at my solution. Here, in a few brief phrases, is the essence of my philosophy:

Make decisions promptly.

Don't agonize over the details of the decision-making process.

Once made, don't rehash decisions.

If a decision is not possible, forget it. Don't dwell on what might have been.

Learn to relax, even in difficult circumstances. Be positive and optimistic.

David Strauss, president, Strauss Construction:

My personal solution as to how I cope with stress in business is that I find I am able to work relatively long hours during the week. For example, I normally work ten hours a day for five days, keeping that pace up for a couple of weeks at a time. Then I try to take an extra day or two off, taking a long weekend to get away and forget about the problems of business. I find that I must really get out of the city, because if I didn't I would find myself working on weekends, which I do not care to do. I also try to work as efficiently as possible in my business, not allowing anything in my personal life to interfere. In this way, I am able to handle a complicated load for brief periods of time.

Franklin D. Murphy, chairman of the board, The Times Mirror Company:

A central factor in dealing with stress is to develop ways to escape it from time to time. For me, this has been mainly involvement in public service activities, primarily art museums and educational institutions. Of course, recreational activities are also helpful. These can be in the form of participation in sports or interest in music, drama, etc. One must have opportunities for intellectual and physical involvement other than those in one's primary job.

The key is not to take work or problems home at night or even over the weekend.

Justin Dart, chairman, Dart Industries:

How do I handle stress? I'm not sure I know.

I think, however, that one learns to live with it. The more experience an individual has with stress and problems, the more easy they are to handle. I think one gets to be a little philosophical about stress. What seems like a tragedy at one period of time doesn't necessarily seem all that bad when it recurs.

Interestingly, and perhaps of no surprise, each executive mentioned sensible distractions, optimism, confidence, and time to relax for prevention of stress. As mentioned in Chapter III, those considered "hardy" view work as a challenge, are strongly committed, and possess a sense of control over their work.

WHAT IS SUCCESS?

Leo Rosten, in a speech entitled "The Free Mind" (delivered in 1962), aptly defined success as follows:

To laugh often and much, to win the respect of people and the affection of children; to earn the appreciation of honest criticism and endure the betrayal of false friends; to appreciate beauty; to find the best in others; to leave the world a bit better, whether by a healthy child, a garden patch or a redeemed social condition; to know even one life has breathed easier because you lived. This is to have succeeded.

Epilogue

In reviewing Dr. Hans Selye's book *Stress Without Distress*, I decided it would be most appropriate to include parts of his last chapter, "Resume," as an epilogue for my book. The following excerpts* summarize his feelings and mine.

Altruistic Egotism

Egotism was the basis of evolution throughout the ages. The originally simplest forms of life, consisting of individual and totally independent cells, were subject to the relentless law of natural selection; those cells that could not protect themselves soon ceased to exist. It also became apparent, however, that such pure egocentricity created dangerous antagonisms, the advantages of one individual often being acquired to the detriment of others. Therefore, a certain degree of altruism had to be introduced for egotistic reasons. Unicellular organisms began to aggregate and form stronger, more complex multicellular beings; in these, certain cells had to give up part of their independence to specialize in nutrition, defense, or locomotion, but thereby the security and survival value of each individual were raised.

Single cells combined into multicellular organisms and these into larger groups on the basis of this principle, although they were not aware of it. Similarly, individual people have formed the cooperative "mutual insurance" groups of the family, tribes, and nations within which altruistic egotism is the key to success. It is the only way to preserve teamwork, whose value is ever increasing in modern society. (pp. 134–135)

---

* Abridged and adapted from Hans Selye, "Stress Without Distress," *School Guidance Worker*, May 1977, quoted with permission of the Guidance Centre, Faculty of Education, University of Toronto, Ontario. Material (as it appeared in *School Guidance Worker*) abridged and adapted from Chapter Five in *Stress Without Distress* by Hans Selye (J. B. Lippincott Company). Copyright © 1974 by Hans Selye, M.D. Reprinted by permission of Harper & Row, Publishers, Inc.

Activity and Diversion

Activity is a biological necessity. We have seen that unused muscles, brains, and other organs lose efficiency. To keep fit, we must exercise both our bodies and our minds. . . . Whether we call our activity exhausting work or relaxing play depends largely upon our own attitude towards it. We should at least get on friendly terms with our job; ideally, we should try to find "play professions" that are pleasant, useful, and constructive as possible. These should give us the best outlets—safety valves—for self-realization, and for preventing irrational violent outbreaks or flight into the dream life of drugs such as occur in people whose high motivation is frustrated by the lack of an acceptable aim. In seeking a worthwhile goal, remember my little jingle: "Fight for your highest attainable aim/but never put up resistance in vain." In other words, it won't hurt you to work hard for something you want, but make sure that it is really you who wants it—not merely your society, parents, teachers, neighbors, "employers"—and that you can be a winner.

As a physician, I have seen innumerable instances of this in patients who suffered from some incapacitating, painful, and incurable disease. Those who sought relief in complete rest suffered most because they could not avoid thinking constantly about their hopeless future, whereas those who managed to go on being active as long as possible gained strength from solving the many little tasks of daily life which took their minds off more sinister considerations. Few things would give more help to the hopeless than to teach them to exploit the healing stress of diversion. (pp. 136–137)

Selye added a prescription for enjoying a full life:

Achieving a Fulfilling Life

We have seen that the stress of frustration is particularly harmful. Man, with his highly developed central nervous system, is especially vulnerable to psychic insults, and there are various little tricks to minimize these. Here are a few that I have found useful:

Even if you systematically want to hoard love, don't waste your time trying to befriend a mad dog.

Admit that there is no perfection, but in each category of achievement something is tops; be satisfied to strive for that.

Do not underestimate the delight of real simplicity in your life style. Avoidance of all affectations and unnecessary complications earns as much goodwill and love as pompous artificiality earns dislike.

Whatever situation you meet in life, consider first whether it is really worth fighting for. Do not forget what Nature has taught us about the importance of carefully adapting . . . to any problems of a cell, a man, or even a society.

Try to keep your mind constantly on the pleasant aspects of life and on actions which can improve your situation. Try to forget everything that is irrevocably ugly or painful. This is perhaps the most efficient way of minimizing stress by what I have called voluntary mental diversion. As a wise German proverb says, "Imitate the sundial's ways;/ Count only the pleasant days."

Nothing paralyzes your efficiency more than frustration; nothing helps it more than success. Even after the greatest defeats the depressing thought of being a failure is best combatted by taking stock of all your past achievements which no one can deny you. Such conscious stock-taking is most effective in re-establishing the self-confidence necessary for future success. There is something even in the most modest career that we are proud to recall—you would be surprised to see how much this can help when everything seems hopeless.

When faced with a task which is very painful yet indispensable to achieve your aim, don't procrastinate; cut right into an abscess to eliminate the pain, instead of prolonging it by gently rubbing the surface.

Realize that men are not created equal, though they should, of course, have a birthright to equal opportunities. After birth, in a free society, their performance should determine their progress. There will always be leaders and followers, but the leaders are worth keeping only as long as they can serve the followers by acquiring their love, respect and gratitude.

Finally, do not forget that there is no ready-made success formula which would suit everybody. We are all different and so are our problems. The only thing we have in common is our subordination to those fundamental biological laws which govern all living beings, including man. Hence, I think a natural code of behavior based on nonspecific mechanisms of adaptation comes closest to what can be offered as a general guideline for conduct. (pp. 141–143)

The following quote cited by Selye might serve as an ideal conclusion for this treatise:

"And one might therefore say of me that in this book I have only made up a bunch of other people's flowers, and that of my own I have only provided the string that ties them together."   —*Montaigne*

Appendices
References
Index

APPENDIX A

The Social Readjustment Rating Scale

As early as the turn of the century, Dr. Adolf Meyer of Johns Hopkins University began investigating the relationship between health and personal crisis. He began keeping charts and biographies of patients. What he found was a dramatic and clear-cut correlation between personal events and disease. Patients who experienced major personal crises frequently became seriously ill within a short period after these events.

Beginning in the 1940s Harold Wolf of Cornell University studied the emotional states and antecedent events that often precede health problems. Thomas H. Holmes also began to apply Meyer's research to over 5,000 case histories and determined that some of these life events appeared over and over again. Years later, Richard H. Rahe studied over 2,000 sailors and found that almost one-third who reported significant life-event changes became ill during their first month at sea. In the sixties researchers Holmes and Rahe (1967) made a significant contribution to the understanding and prevention of stressful life events. The life events that appear in their Social Readjustment Rating Scale,* as shown below, include both positive and negative factors. The number assigned to each event is a weight determined by statistical analysis. Each item was found to create upheaval in one's life, thus causing bodily readjustment in a large sample of people. Review the list and add up your sum based upon the changes that have occurred in the previous year.

* Reprinted with permission from *Journal of Psychosomatic Research*, 11, T. H. Holmes and R. H. Rahe, "The Social Readjustment Rating Scale." Copyright 1967, Pergamon Press, Ltd.

THE SOCIAL READJUSTMENT RATING SCALE

Life Event	*Mean Value*
1. Death of spouse	100
2. Divorce	73
3. Marital separation	65
4. Jail term	63
5. Death of close family member	63
6. Personal injury or illness	53
7. Marriage	50
8. Fired at work	47
9. Marital reconciliation	45
10. Retirement	45
11. Change in health of family member	44
12. Pregnancy	40
13. Sex difficulties	39
14. Gain of new family member	39
15. Business readjustment	39
16. Change in financial state	38
17. Death of close friend	37
18. Change to different line of work	36
19. Change in number of arguments with spouse	35
20. Mortgage over $10,000	31
21. Foreclosure of mortgage or loan	30
22. Change in responsibilities at work	29
23. Son or daughter leaving home	29
24. Trouble with in-laws	29
25. Outstanding personal achievement	28
26. Wife begins or stops work	26
27. Begin or end of school	26
28. Change in living conditions	25
29. Revision of personal habits	24
30. Trouble with boss	23
31. Change in work hours or conditions	20
32. Change in residence	20
33. Change in schools	20
34. Change in recreation	19
35. Change in church activities	19
36. Change in social activities	18
37. Mortgage or loan less than $10,000	17
38. Change in sleeping habits	16
39. Change in number of family get-togethers	15

Life Event	Mean Value
40. Change in eating habits	15
41. Vacation	13
42. Christmas	12
43. Minor violations of the law	11

The more changes one undergoes in a 12-month period of time, the more points one accumulates. A score of 150–199 = safe ground (10–30 percent chance of serious health change), 200+ = moderate ground (30–50 percent chance of serious health change), 300+ = serious ground (50–90 percent chance of serious health change), 450+ = standing on earthquake fault (90 percent chance of serious health change).

It is important to emphasize that the percentages are probabilities and not inevitabilities. A high score may serve as a significant warning to review current life events and creatively avoid future distress.

You Possess
Type A Behavior Pattern

Meyer Friedman, M.D. and Ray H. Rosenman, M.D. (1974) developed this list of type A characteristics. How many of them do you have?

1. If you have (a) a habit of explosively accentuating various key words in your ordinary speech even when there is no real need for such accentuation, and (b) a tendency to utter the last few words of your sentences far more rapidly than the opening words. The vocal explosiveness betrays the excess aggression or hostility you may be harboring. The hurrying of the ends of sentences mirrors your underlying impatience with spending even the time required for your own speech.

2. If you always move, walk, and eat rapidly.

3. If you feel (particularly if you openly exhibit to others) an impatience with the rate at which most events take place. You are suffering from this sort of impatience if you find it difficult to restrain yourself from hurrying the speech of others and resort to the device of saying very quickly over and over again, "Uh huh, uh huh," or, "Yes yes, yes yes," to someone who is talking, unconsciously urging him to "get on with" or hasten his rate of speaking. You are also suffering from impatience if you attempt

to finish the sentences of persons speaking to you before they can. Other signs of this sort of impatience: if you become unduly irritated or even enraged when a car ahead of you in your lane runs at a pace you consider too slow; if you find it anguishing to wait in a line or to wait your turn to be seated at a restaurant; if you find it intolerable to watch others perform tasks you know you can do faster; if you become impatient with yourself as you are obliged to perform repetitious duties (making out bank deposit slips, writing checks, washing and cleaning dishes, and so on), which are necessary but take you away from doing things you really have an interest in doing; if you find yourself hurrying your own reading or always attempting to obtain condensations or summaries of truly interesting and worthwhile literature.

4. If you indulge in polyphasic thought or performance, frequently striving to think of or do two or more things simultaneously. For example, if while trying to listen to another person's speech you persist in continuing to think about an irrelevant subject, you are indulging in polyphasic thought. Similarly, if while golfing or fishing you continue to ponder your business or professional problems, or if while using an electric razor you attempt also to eat your breakfast or drive your car, or if while driving your car you attempt to dictate letters for your secretary, you are indulging in polyphasic performance. This is one of the commonest traits in the Type A man. Nor is he always satisfied with doing just two things at one time. We have known subjects who not only shaved and ate simultaneously, but also managed to read a business or professional journal at the same time.

5. If you find it always difficult to refrain from talking about or bringing the theme of any conversation around to those subjects which especially interest and intrigue you, and when unable to accomplish this maneuver, you pretend to listen but really remain preoccupied with your own thoughts.

6. If you almost always feel vaguely guilty when you relax and do absolutely nothing for several hours to several days.

7. If you no longer observe the more important or interesting or lovely objects that you encounter in your milieu. For example, if you enter a strange office, store, or home and after leaving any of these places you cannot recall what was in them, you no longer are observing well—or for that matter enjoying life very much.

8. If you do not have any time to spare to become the things worth being because you are so preoccupied with getting the things worth having.

9. If you attempt to schedule more and more in less and less time, and in doing so make fewer and fewer allowances for unforeseen contingencies. A concomitant of this is a chronic sense of time urgency, one of the core components of Type A Behavior Pattern.

10. If, on meeting another severely afflicted Type A person, instead of feeling compassion for his affliction you find yourself compelled to "challenge" him. This is a telltale trait because no one arouses the aggressive and/or hostile feelings of one Type A subject more quickly than another Type A subject.

11. If you resort to certain characteristic gestures or nervous tics. For example, if in conversation you frequently clench your fist, or bang your hand upon a table or pound one fist into the palm of your other hand in order to emphasize a conversational point, you are exhibiting Type A gestures. Similarly, if the corners of your mouth spasmodically, in tic-like fashion, jerk backward slightly exposing your teeth, you are subject to muscular phenomena suggesting the presence of a continuous struggle, which is, of course, the kernel of the Type A Behavior Pattern.

12. If you believe that whatever success you have enjoyed has been due in good part to your ability to get things done faster than your fellow men and if you are afraid to stop doing everything faster and faster.

13. If you find yourself increasingly and reluctantly committed to translating and evaluating not only your own but also the activities of others in terms of "numbers."

In summary, a Type A individual: is characterized by frenzied speed in moving, talking, and eating; hates lines or drinking slowly; schedules more activities than time is available for; loathes "wasting" time; becomes impatient with others' perceived slowness; has little if any time available for intimacy, relaxation, or enjoyment; and never seems to catch up.

How Well Can You Relax?

	Always	Sometimes	Seldom
1. Are you able to shut out your worries when you go to bed at night?	___	___	___
2. Are you able to take a nap during the day and awaken refreshed?	___	___	___
3. Is your clothing well fitting and relaxing?	___	___	___
4. Are you able to concentrate on one problem at a time?	___	___	___
5. Do you plan your day's activities?	___	___	___
6. Do you find time to relax and stretch during the day?	___	___	___
7. Do you schedule a certan portion of each day as uninterruptible?	___	___	___
8. When you feel yourself becoming tense because of sustained positions, do you know how to relax by doing simple exercises or activities?	___	___	___
9. Do you check yourself frequently for habitual tension habits, such as scowling, clenched fists, tight jaws, hunched shoulders, or pursed lips?	___	___	___
10. Do you relax these evidences of tension at will when you find them?	___	___	___
11. Do you find it easy to relax so that you sleep easily and deeply?	___	___	___
12. Do you know how to release ten-			

Adapted by Gmelch (1977) from Janet Wessel, *Movement Fundamentals* (New York: Prentice-Hall, 1957), p. 55. Used by permission of Janet Wessel.

Always   *Sometimes*   *Seldom*

sions through simple movements so
that you can sleep well?   _____   _____   _____

13. Do you play with such interest that
you become completely absorbed in
what you are doing?   _____   _____   _____

14. Do you plan your life to have a
change of people, scenery, and
thoughts?   _____   _____   _____

TOTAL NUMBER MARKED:

Always _____   Sometimes _____   Seldom _____

RATING: SCORE:

Always—3 points   33–42 points—high ability to relax
Sometimes—2 points   24–32 points—average ability to relax
Seldom—1 point   15–23 points—low ability to relax

Suggestions for Education

Andrew J. DuBrin ("Teacher Burnout," 1979b), industrial psychologist at the University of Rochester, claims that some teachers don't know how to play the school politics game. Here are 12 temptations DuBrin finds that many otherwise sensible teachers seem unable to resist.* Succumbing to them results in alienation from administrators and colleagues and immeasurable stress.

- Badmouthing other teachers or administrators to the public or, worse, to your students. Word of such indiscretions usually gets back to the offended parties. The result: a climate of ill will.
- Creating unpleasant surprises for your principal. Life is difficult enough for most principals. If you know a parent is preparing a lawsuit, inform the administration.
- Going out of your way to file grievances. Few people enjoy being around ingrates or malcontents. Why file a grievance just because one meeting runs 30 minutes late?
- Running around your principal to bring some matter to the attention of your superintendent. For example, bypassing your principal to get a physical education dispensation for a student communicates your message: "I don't think my principal is very effective."
- Making picky little demands. Most administrators abhor such unprofessional behavior as insuring that all your sick days are used each year. Many of your peers feel the same way when you take eight sick days in May.
- Complaining at a PTA meeting that new developments in education are hurting teaching. Saying to a parent, "We would have more

---

money for salaries if we didn't spend so much money on junk like teaching machines" creates tension between the principal and public.

- Being the informal leader of a group of malcontents among your colleagues. It may be morally important for you to do so; but recognize that such an action automatically alienates you.
- Making derogatory comments about problem students to other teachers. Many of your peers are parents themselves. Might you also refer to their child as a "miserable little psychopath?"
- Bragging about your outside business. Stating that your family restaurant, for example, is doing so well that soon you will be able to quit teaching is stomping on the toes of peers who choose to remain in teaching.
- Grumbling because you spent five dollars out-of-pocket for school supplies. Instead, claim that five dollars as a professional expense when you file your income tax!
- Insisting that nobody with good sense would enter the field of education these days. Why spread your demoralized feelings?
- Violating the dress code. Sure, it's your constitutional right to wear almost any clothing to work. But some administrators take it personally, feeling it an act of defiance against them.

APPENDIX E

A Teacher's Ten Commandments

What do veteran teachers do to keep fresh, excited, and wide-eyed about teaching? Peggie Case Paulus ("Teacher Burnout," 1979b) suggests these ten commandments.* Raise your right hand and read aloud:

    I. Keep alert to changing methods and philosophies.
   II. Attend conferences, workshops, and in-service programs with an open mind.
  III. Listen to other teachers in your school.
  IV. Avoid like the plague the stereotype of talking only about school after hours.
    V. Keep alert physically and mentally.
  VI. Keep in step with students and find out about their hobbies, movies, and music.
 VII. Discard . . . discard . . . discard old ideas, old prejudices, old materials.
VIII. Read more than "Dick and Jane" books and subscribe to professional magazines.
  IX. Be flexible and avoid doing something just because it's always been done that way.
   X. Keep your senses sharpened, your mind keen, and your heart open to remain an enthusiastic teacher!

---

* Reprinted and adapted from *Instructor,* January 1979, p. 59. Copyright © 1979 by The Instructor Publications, Inc. Used by permission.

A Healthy, Well-adjusted Person

In order to better understand the goal of effective personal development, one must be aware of the differences between healthy and unhealthy individuals. The behavioral characteristics of a *healthy* individual include:

- The ability to make judgments or attempt something new without regret, guilt, or fear of disapproval.
- Having the confidence to deal with problems even when failure might occur.
- Celebrating one's failures as necessary in learning.
- Valuing and having a genuine interest in others.
- Accepting praise and compliments without embarrassment.
- Resisting others' attempts to dominate oneself.
- Feeling equal rather than inferior or superior to others.
- Thinking and acting spontaneously, but accepting the conventional in order to avoid hurting others.
- Seeing reality as it is and being comfortable in relationship to it (less wishful thinking, e.g., "If only I . . .").
- Accepting the fact that on various occasions, one feels a wide range of socially acceptable and unacceptable impulses.
- Being self-reliant by solving most problems on one's own, although not being afraid to ask for ideas or help.
- Acknowledging and taking personal responsibility for one's actions.
- Needing some time for solitude and privacy without feeling discomfort or emptiness.
- Gaining pleasure each day from the beauty of one's life and environment.

- Having the ability to learn from beliefs and ideas similar and different from one's own.
- Having an unhostile, spontaneous sense of humor that laughs *with*, not *at* others.
- Being able to find some aspect of behavior in oneself that is not liked and setting out to change it.

Eupsychian Management

The following assumptions underlie Eupsychian Management policy, espoused by Abraham Maslow.*

1. Assume everyone is to be trusted.
2. Assume everyone is to be informed as completely as possible of as many facts and truths as possible, i.e., everything relevant to the situation.
3. Assume in your people the impulse to achieve.
4. Assume that there is no dominance-subordination hierarchy in the jungle sense or authoritarian sense.
5. Assume that everyone will have the same ultimate managerial objectives and will identify with them no matter where they are in the organization or in the hierarchy.
6. Eupsychian economics must assume good will among all the members of the organization rather than rivalry or jealousy.
7. Assume that the individuals involved are healthy enough.
8. Assume that the organization is healthy enough, whatever this means.
9. Assume the ability to admire, i.e., to be objective and detached.
10. We must assume the people are not fixated at the safety-need level.
11. Assume an active trend to self-actualization.
12. Assume that everyone can enjoy good teamwork, friendship, good group spirit, good homogeny, good belongingness and group love.
13. Assume hostility to be primarily reactive rather than character-based.

---

* Abridged from Abraham H. Maslow, *Eupsychian Management: A Journal* (Homewood, Ill.: Richard D. Irwin and The Dorsey Press, 1965), pp. 17–33. © 1965 by Richard D. Irwin, Inc. Reprinted by permission.

14. Assume that people can take it, that they are tough, stronger than most people give them credit for.
15. Eupsychian management assumes that people are improvable.
16. Assume that everyone prefers to feel important, needed, useful, successful, proud, respected, rather than unimportant, interchangeable, anonymous, wasted, unused, expendable and disrespected.
17. Assume that everyone prefers or even needs to love his boss (rather than to hate him), and that everyone prefers to respect his boss (rather than to disrespect him).
18. Assume that everyone dislikes fearing anyone, but that he prefers fearing the boss to despising him.
19. Assume that everyone prefers to be a prime mover rather than a passive helper.
20. Assume a tendency to improve things, to straighten the crooked picture on the wall, to clean up the dirty mess, to put things right, make things better and to do things better.
21. Assume that growth occurs through delight and not through boredom.
22. Assume preference for being a whole person and not a part, not a thing or an implement, or tool, or "hand."
23. Assume the preference for working rather than being idle.
24. All human beings, not only Eupsychian ones, prefer meaningful work to meaningless work.
25. Assume the preference for personhood, uniqueness as a person, identity.
26. We must make the assumption that the person is courageous enough for Eupsychian processes.
27. We must make the specific assumptions of nonpsychopathy.
28. We must assume the wisdom and the efficacy of self-choice.
29. We must assume that everyone likes to be justly and fairly appreciated, preferably in public.
30. We must assume the defense and growth dialectic for all these positive trends that we have listed above.
31. Assume that everyone but especially the more developed persons prefer responsibility to dependency and passivity most of the time.
32. The general assumption is that people will get more pleasure out of loving than they will out of hating.
33. Assume that fairly well-developed people would rather create than destroy.
34. Assume that fairly well-developed people would rather be interested than bored.

Why It Won't Work

Below is a ready-reference list of reasons why "it won't work," applicable to any suggested changes in education (tongue in cheek).

1. We tried that before.
2. Our place is different.
3. It costs too much.
4. That's beyond our responsibility.
5. That's not my job.
6. We're all too busy to do that.
7. It's too radical a change.
8. We don't have the time.
9. Not enough help.
10. That will make other equipment obsolete.
11. Let's make a research test of it first.
12. Our school is too small for it.
13. Not practical for teachers (students, principals, etc.).
14. The parents will never buy it.
15. The union will scream.
16. We've never done it before.
17. It's against school policy.
18. Runs up our overhead.
19. We don't have the authority.
20. That's too ivory tower.
21. That's not our problem.
22. Let's get back to reality.
23. Why change it, it's still working O.K.
24. I don't like the idea.
25. You're right, but . . .

26. You're two years ahead of your time.
27. We're not ready for that.
28. We don't have the money, equipment, personnel.
29. It isn't in the budget.
30. Can't teach an old dog new tricks.
31. Good enough, but impractical.
32. Let's hold it in abeyance.
33. Let's give it more thought.
34. The school board will never go for it.
35. Let's put it in writing.
36. We'll be the laughing stock.
37. Not *that* again!
38. We'd lose money in the long run.
39. Where'd you dig that one up?
40. We did all right without it.
41. It's never been tried before.
42. Let's shelve it for the time being.
43. Has anyone else ever tried it?
44. Let's form a committee.
45. I don't see the connection.
46. What you are really saying is . . .
47. Maybe that will work in your department . . . but in mine . . .
48. I know a fellow who tried it.
49. Let's all sleep on it.
50. We've always done it this way.

APPENDIX I

Memorable Quotes

Over a period of years I have collected many memorable quotes. Some are from noted authors, others from unknown writers. They can provide meaning and inner strength, and serve as truly enjoyable mental diversions. When stress begins to turn to distress, a few well-chosen lines can have a significant impact.

It is not doing what you like, but in liking what you do that is the secret of happiness. *Sir James Barrie*

Following the path of least resistance is what makes men and rivers crooked. *Voltaire*

I shall pass through this world but once. Any good that I can do, or any kindness that I can show any human being, let me do it now and not deter it. For I shall not pass this way again. *Stephen Grellet*

Experience is what you get when you were expecting something else. *Marvin G. Gregory*

When change is successful we call it growth. *Anonymous*

You can make more friends in two months by becoming really interested in other people, than you can in two years by trying to get other people interested in you. *Dale Carnegie*

You can tell more about a person by what he says about others than you can by what others say about him. *Marvin G. Gregory*

If you think you're confused, consider poor Columbus. He didn't know where he was going; when he got there, he didn't know where he was; and when he got back, he didn't know where he'd been. *Anonymous*

A fault recognized is half corrected.   *Old Proverb*

The mind is like a parachute. It only works when it's open.
                                                      Rollie Katz

It is sometimes better to keep your mouth shut and let people think you're a fool, than to open it and remove all doubt.   *Mark Twain*

Man is the only animal that laughs and weeps; for man is the only animal that perceives how things are and how they ought to be.
                                                      William Hazlitt

If there was nothing that men desired more than life, would they not use any possible means of preserving it? And if there was more than death, would they not do anything to escape from danger? Yet there are means of preserving one's life which men will not use, ways of avoiding danger which men will not adopt. Thus it appears that men desire some things more than life, and hate some things more than death.   *Mencius*

Yesterday is already a dream and tomorrow is only a vision, but today well lived makes every yesterday a dream of happiness and every tomorrow a vision of hope.   *Sanskrit Proverb*

Take time to think, It is the source of power.
Take time to play, It is the secret of perpetual youth.
Take time to read, It is the fountain of wisdom.
Take time to hope, It is the greatest potential on earth.
Take time to love and be loved, It is a nourishment of life.
Take time to be friendly, It is the road to happiness.
Take time to laugh, It is the music of the soul.
Take time to give, It is too short a day to be selfish.
Take time to work, It is the price of success.
                                                      Anonymous

Most people are just about as happy as they make up their minds to be.   *Abraham Lincoln*

Don't be afraid to take a big step if one is indicated. You can't cross a chasm in two small jumps.   *Anonymous*

Children of today love luxury. They have bad manners, contempt for authority and they show disrespect for their elders. They no longer show manners when elders enter the room. They contradict their parents, continually chatter, gobble up things and tyrannize their teachers.   *Socrates*

Financial success is purely metallic. The man who gains it has four metallic attributes: gold in his palm, silver on his tongue, brass on his face, and iron in his heart.   *Abraham Lincoln*

The more we study the more we discover our ignorance.
                                                                                Percy Bysshe Shelley

Sometimes a fool has talent but never judgment.   *La Rochefoucauld*

Learning makes a man fit company for himself.   *Edward Young*

Husband to wife: I liked the old educational system better—when they disciplined the child instead of lecturing the parents.
                                                                                        Anonymous

If a man does not keep pace with his companions, perhaps it is because he hears a different drummer. Let him step to the music which he hears, however measured or far away.   *Henry David Thoreau*

A good teacher is one who can understand those who are not very good at explaining, and explain to those who are not very good at understanding.   *Dwight D. Eisenhower*

Let the dead past bury its dead. The load of tomorrow, added to that of yesterday carried today make the strongest falter. Shut off the future as tightly as the past. The future is today, close then the great fore and aft bulkheads and prepare to cultivate the habit of a life of day-tight compartments.   *Sir William Osler*

Anyone can do his work however hard for one day. Anyone can live sweetly, patiently, lovingly, purely till the sun goes down. And this is all that life really means.   *Robert Louis Stevenson*

Life is too short to be little.   *Benjamin Disraeli*

There is only one way to happiness and that is to cease worrying about things which are beyond the power of our will.   *Epictetus*

When you are good to others, you are best to yourself.
                                                                                Benjamin Franklin

I never did a day's work in life. It was all fun.   *Thomas A. Edison*

Perhaps the most valuable result of all education is the ability to make yourself do the thing you have to do when it ought to be done, whether you like it or not; it is the first lesson that ought to be learned; and however early a man's training begins, it is probably the last lesson that he learns thoroughly.   *Thomas Huxley*

Whenever you can save some of your time by offering money in its place, do so. Strangely, from their earliest beginnings men have always seemed quite happy to trade the very limited days of their lives for discs of copper, bronze, silver, and gold.
Meyer Friedman, M.D., and Ray H. Rosenman, M.D.

It is more important to do the right thing than to do things right.
Peter Drucker

The secret of being miserable is to have the leisure to bother about whether you are happy or not. *George Bernard Shaw*

The ancestor of every action is a thought. *Ralph Waldo Emerson*

Tension is a habit. Relaxation is a habit, and bad habits can be broken and good habits formed. *William James*

The Unknown Teacher
I sing the praises of the Unknown Teacher. Great generals win campaigns but it is the Unknown Soldier who wins the war. Famous educators plan new systems of pedagogy, but it is the Unknown Teacher who delivers and guides the young. He lives in obscurity and contends with hardship. For him, no trumpets blare, no chariots wait, no golden decorations are decreed. He keeps the watch along the borders of darkness and makes the attack on the trenches of ignorance and folly. Patient in his duty, he strives to conquer the evil powers which are enemies of youth. He awakens sleeping spirits. He quickens the indolent, encourages the eager, and steadies the unstable. He communicates his own joy in learning, and shares with boys and girls the best treasures of his mind. He lights many candles, which in later years, will shine back to cheer him. This is his reward. No one is more worthy to be enrolled in a democratic aristocracy, king of himself, and servant of mankind. *Henry Van Dyke*

The most important thing in life is not to capitalize on your gains. Any fool can do that. The really important thing is to profit from your losses. That requires intelligence, and it makes the difference between a man of sense and a fool. *William Bolitho*

Most of the shadows of this life are caused by standing in one's own sunshine. *Ralph Waldo Emerson*

The lowest ebb is the turn of the tide.
Henry Wadsworth Longfellow

This above all, to thine own self be true,
And it must follow as the night the day
Thou canst not then be false to any man.

William Shakespeare

God, grant me the serenity to accept the things I cannot change; the courage to change the things I can; and the wisdom to know the difference.   *Attributed by Dale Carnegie to Reinhold Niebuhr*

Each moment of the year has its own beauty which was never seen before and which never will be seen again.   *Ralph Waldo Emerson*

The trouble with being an educational leader today is that you can't be sure whether people are following you or chasing you.

Anonymous

Life is a banquet and most damn fools are starving to death.

Auntie Mame

Work is love made visible.   *Kahlil Gibran*

I Am The Child
I am the child
All the world waits for my coming.
All the earth watches with interest to see what I shall become.
Civilization hangs in the balance.
For what I am the world of tomorrow will be.
I am the child.
I have come into your world, about which I knew nothing.
Why I came I know not.
How I came I know not.
I am curious; I am interested.
I am the child.
You hold in your hand my destiny.
You determine largely whether I shall succeed or fail.
Give me, I pray you, those things that make for happiness.
Train me, I beg you, that I may be a blessing to this world.

Mamie Cole

All of us are the children of condition, of circumstances, of environment, of education, of acquired habits, and of heredity, molding men as they are and will forever be.   *Abraham Lincoln*

I am going to meet people today who talk too much—people who are selfish, egotistical, ungrateful. But, I won't be surprised or disturbed for I couldn't imagine a world without such people.

Marcus Aurelius

Hate is like acid. It can damage the vessel in which it is stored as well as destroy the object on which it is poured.   *Ann Landers*

Better take an interest in the future; you're going to spend the rest of your life there.
Anonymous

A sorrow shared is but half a trouble
But a joy that's shared is made double.

Old Proverb

Happiness makes up in height what it lacks in length.   *Robert Frost*

Knowledge is proud that he has learned so much,
wisdom is humble that he knows no more.

William Cooper

I am indebted to my father for living but to my teacher for living well.   *Alexander of Macedon*

Arrogance, pedantry and dogmatism are the occupational diseases of those who spend their lives directing the intellects of the young.
Henry Seidel Canby

It is by education I learn to do by choice what other men do by constraint of fear.   *Aristotle*

Our wretched species is so made that those who walk on the well-trodden path always throw stones at those who are showing a new road.
Voltaire

The surest way to corrupt a youth is to instruct him to hold in higher esteem those who think alike than those who think differently.

Friedrich Nietzsche

A person's a person, no matter how small.
from HORTON HEARS A WHO by *Dr. Seuss*

Children have more need of models than critics.   *Joseph Joubert*

We must stop fragmenting children! Learning-disabled children, like Humpty Dumpty, need to be put together.   *Margaret Mutti*

Grown-ups are in such a hurry but "It takes a lot of slow to grow."
Eve Merriam

Don't be afraid to try something *new*, Joey. I thought carrots were terrible until I tasted sauerkraut.
from DENNIS THE MENACE by *Hank Ketcham*

The trick, Fletcher, is that we are trying to overcome our limitations in order, patiently. We don't tackle flying through rock until a little later in the program.

from JONATHAN LIVINGSTON SEAGULL by *Richard Bach*

It may be true that the weak will always be driven to the wall; but it is the task of society to see that the wall is climbable.

Sydney Harris

A teacher affects eternity.   *Henry Adams*

Look forward to the Butterfly instead of stepping on the Caterpillar.

Eleanor Wynne

The happiness of life is made up of the little charities of a kiss or smile, a kind look, a heartfelt compliment.   *Samuel Taylor Coleridge*

When your only tool is a hammer you go about treating everything as a nail.   *Abraham Maslow*

We must learn to live together as brothers or perish together as fools.

Martin Luther King

Please remind them that time is short.

Aldous Huxley (on his deathbed)

After you understand all about the sun and the stars, and rotation of the earth, you may still miss the radiance of the sunset.

Alfred North Whitehead

To me every hour of the day and night is an unspeakably perfect miracle.   *Walt Whitman*

It is wiser to choose what you say than to say what you choose.

Harold Hayden

Factors of Job Stress

The following factors were adapted from Beehr and Newman (1978) and represent those identified as contributory to job stress.*

Occupational Environment Factors

weekly work schedule†
over and under-utilization of skills†
variance in work load
pace of work
responsibility (for people or things)
travel as part of the job
job characteristics considered intrinsically motivating
role overload†
role ambiguity†
formal and informal relationships among organizational members
size of organization†
job security
hours of work (both total and time of day)†
duration of work tasks
sociotechnical changes
organizational structure (and job position within hierarchy)
communication system (and job position within system)†
organizational policies and procedures
management style (philosophical and operational)†
evaluation and reward systems
training programs†

---

* Adapted from T. Beehr and N. Newman, "Job Stress, Employee Health, and Organizational Effectiveness: A Facet Analysis, Model, and Literature Review," *Personnel Psychology,* 1978, 3, 665–699. Used by permission.
† Factors where extensive empirical study has been conducted.

organizational climate
opportunity for advancement
required relocation
local union constraints
perceptions of clients
route to and from work
number and nature of clients
governmental laws and regulations
suppliers; providers of needed services
weather
technological and scientific developments
consumer movements
geographic location of organization

Personal Factors

psychological condition (personality traits and behavioral characteristics, for example, need for clarity/intolerance of ambiguity)†
"Type A" personality†
approval-seeking
defensiveness
impatience
intrapersonal conflicts (between ego-ideal and reality)
self-esteem
career and life motives/goals/aspirations
anxiety level
perceptual style
values (human, religious)
personal work standards
need for perfection
intelligence†
abilities (especially task and coping-related)
previous experience with stress
satisfaction with job and other major aspects of life
physical fitness/health†
diet and eating habits
exercise, work, sleep, and relaxation patterns†
family stages
career stages
age†
education (amount and type)†
sex†
race
socioeconomic status

The School Administrator's Job

The school administrator's job involves at least the following tasks:*

Evaluation
Conferencing
Reports
Communication
District, State, and Federal
    Legal Requirements
Supervision
Curriculum
Fiscal
Advisory/Site Council
Pupil Assessment
Program Assessment
Ongoing Planning
Staff Development
Physical Plant
Intergroup Conflict
Exclusive Bargaining Contract
Cafeteria
Negotiations
Instructional Materials
Civic Center

Co-Curricular
Categorical Aid
Meetings
Selection of Staff
Student Discipline
Safety
Health Services
Attendance
Master Planning—Special Educa-
    tion
Community Participation
Student Supervision
Scheduling
Temporary Employees
Student Transportation
Emergency Procedures
District Support Personnel
Student Achievement
Population Shifts
Transience
Interpersonal Relationships

* This matrix was included in a special report by the Association of California School Administrators (ACSA), "Changing Role of the Principal," Sacramento, May 1978.

Planning for Change
Follow-Up of Students
Public Relations
Special Programs
Professional Growth
Organizational Structure
Decision-Making Participation
Management of Contractual Obligation

Emergencies
Summer School
Distribution of Authority
Visitors
Fund Raising
Student Activities
Pupil Personnel Services
Pupil Records
Field Trips
Directory Information

Recommended Literature

Albrecht, K. *Stress and the manager.* Englewood Cliffs, N.J.: Prentice-Hall, 1979.

Benson, H. *The relaxation response.* New York: Morrow, 1975.

Bloomfield, H., Cain, M., & Joffe, D. *TM: Discovering inner energy and overcoming stress.* New York: Delacorte Press, 1975.

Carnegie, D. *How to stop worrying and start living.* New York: Simon & Schuster, 1944.

Carruthers, M. *The western way of death: Stress, tension, and heart attacks.* New York: Pantheon, 1974.

Dyer, W. *Your erroneous zones!* New York: Crowell, 1976.

Freudenberger, H. Burn out: Occupational hazard of the child care worker. *Child Care Quarterly,* 1977, *6,* 90–99.

Friedman, M., & Rosenman, R. *Type A behavior and your heart.* New York: Knopf, 1974.

Glasser, W. *Positive addiction.* New York: Harper & Row, 1976.

Greenberg, H. *Coping with job stress.* Englewood Cliffs, N.J.: Prentice-Hall, 1980.

Holmes, T., & Rahe, R. The social readjustment scale. *Journal of Psychosomatic Medicine,* 1967, *11,* 213–218.

Jacobson, E. *You must relax* (5th ed.). New York: McGraw-Hill, 1978.

Lakein, A. *How to take control of your time and life.* New York: Signet, 1973.

Lamott, K. *Escape from stress: How to stop killing yourself.* New York: Putnam, 1974.

McGrath, J. *Social and psychological factors in stress.* New York: Holt, Rinehart & Winston, 1970.

McGregor, D. *The human side of enterprise.* New York: McGraw-Hill, 1960.

McLean, A. *Occupational stress*. Springfield, Ill.: Charles C. Thomas, 1974.

Maslach, C. Burned-out. *Human Behavior*, 1976, 5, 16–22.

Mattingly, M. Sources of stress and burn-out in professional child care work. *Child Care Quarterly*, 1977, 6, 100–113.

Meichenbaum, D. *Cognitive behavior modification*. New York: Plenum Press, 1977.

Pembrook, L. *How to beat fatigue*. Garden City, N.Y.: Doubleday, 1974.

Schafer, W. *Stress, distress, and growth*. Davis, Calif.: Responsible Action, 1978.

Selye, H. *The stress of life* (2nd ed.). New York: McGraw-Hill, 1976.

Selye, H. *Stress without distress*. New York: Lippincott, 1974.

Spaniol, L., & Caputo, J. *Professional burnout: A personal survival kit*. Lexington, Mass.: Human Services Associates, 1979.

Teacher burnout: A national issue says NEA panel. *NEA Reporter*, October 1979, p. 7.

Truch, S. *Teacher burnout*. Novato, Calif.: Academic Therapy Publications, 1980.

Woolfolk, R., & Richardson, F. *Stress, sanity and survival*. New York: Monarch, 1978.

Yates, J. *Managing stress*. New York: AMACOM, 1979.

References

Abdel-Halim, A. Employee affective responses to organizational stress: Moderating effects of job characteristics. *Personnel Psychology*, 1978, *31*, 561–579.

Adams, J. Guidelines for stress management and life style changes. *Personnel Administrator*, 1979, *24*, 35–44.

Albrecht, K. *Stress and the manager.* Englewood Cliffs, N.J.: Prentice-Hall, 1979.

Aldridge, J. Emotional illness and the work environment. *Ergonomics*, 1970, *13*, 613–621.

Alschuler, A., & Shea, J. The discipline game: Playing without losers. *Learning*, August/September 1974, pp. 80–86.

Amato, T., Baird, J., Jackson, W., Johnson, R., Matthews, M., & Thayer, A. The changing role of the principal. Association of California School Administrators Report (first draft). April 1978.

Argyris, C. *Management and organizational development.* New York: McGraw-Hill, 1971.

Askins, J. Beating the 9–5 grind. *San Jose Mercury News*, July 1, 1979, pp. 1L, 6L.

Association of California School Administrators. Changing role of the principal (special report). Sacramento, May 1978.

Beck, A. Cognitive therapy: Nature and relation to behavior therapy. *Behavior Therapy*, 1970, *1*, 184–200.

Beehr, T., & Newman, N. Job stress, employee health, and organizational effectiveness: A facet analysis, model, and literature review. *Personnel Psychology*, 1978, *31*, 665–699.

Belloc, N. Relationship of health practices and mortality. *Preventive Medicine*, 1973, *2*, 67–81.

Bennis, W. Leadership theory and administration: The problem of authority. *Administrative Science Quarterly*, 1959, *4*, 259–301.

Bennis, W. *Changing organizations.* New York: McGraw-Hill, 1966.

Bennis, W. Beyond bureaucracy. In W. Bennis & P. Slater (Eds.), *The temporary society*. New York: Harper & Row, 1968.

Benson, H. *The relaxation response*. New York: Morrow, 1975.

Berry, D. Career planning—You can get there from here. *Manage*, 1977, *29*, 15–17.

Bishop, J. Age of anxiety. *Wall Street Journal*, April 2, 1979, p. 26.

Bloomfield, H. *TM: Discovering inner energy and overcoming stress*. New York: Dell, 1975.

Breslow, L., & Buell, P. Mortality from coronary heart disease and physical activity of work in California. *Journal of Chronic Disorders*, 1960, *11*, 615–626.

Brown, F. Job satisfaction of educational administrators: A replication. *Planning and Changing*, 1976, *7*, 45–53.

Bryan, W. Preventing burnout in the public interest community. *The Grantsmanship Center News*, March/April 1981, pp. 15–75.

Buck, V. *Working under pressure*. London: Staples, 1972.

Burgoyne, J. Stress motivation and learning. In D. Gowler & K. Legge (Eds.), *Managerial stress*. New York: Halstead Press, 1975.

Burns, T., & Stalker, G. *The management of innovation*. London: Tavistock, 1961.

Calamidas, A. Distress and burnout will kill productivity. *Pennsylvania State University Continuing Education News*. State College, Pa.: Management Development Services, 1979(a).

Calamidas, A. Personal communication, 1979(b).

California School Boards Association (CSBA). *Indepth*, Special Financial Issue, Feb./March 1981.

California State Department of Education, Office of Program and Evaluation, *School effectiveness study: The first year*. Sacramento: The Department, 1977.

Cannon, W. *The wisdom of the body*. New York: Norton, 1932.

Caplan, R. Organizational stress and individual strain. Unpublished doctoral dissertation, University of Michigan, Ann Arbor, 1971.

Caplan, R., Cobb, S., French, J., Harrison, R., & Pinneau, S. *Job demands and worker health: Main effects and occupational differences* (HEW Publication No. 75–160, National Institute for Occupational Safety & Health). Washington, D.C.: U.S. Government Printing Office, 1975.

Caplan, R., & Jones, K. Effects of workload, role ambiguity and type A personality on anxiety, depression and heart rate. *Journal of Applied Psychology*, 1975, *60*, 713–719.

Carnegie, D. *How to stop worrying and start living*. New York: Simon and Schuster, 1944.

Cassel, J. The contribution of the social environment to host resistance. *American Journal of Epidemiology*, 1976, *104*, 107–123.

Cedoline, A. A study of the Oak Grove School District administrators. Unpublished paper. San Jose, Calif., June 1979.

Cedoline, A. A comparison between education and fourteen major industries in Santa Clara County. Unpublished paper. San Jose, Calif., June 1980.

Chatfield-Taylor, J. Job burnout. *San Francisco Chronicle*, July 13, 1979, p. 28.

Cherniss, C., Egnatios, E., & Wacker, S. Job stress and career development in new public professionals. *Professional Psychology*, 1976, *24*, 428–436.

Coates, T., & Thoresen, C. Teacher anxiety: A review with recommendations. Stanford, Calif.: Stanford Center for Research and Development, April 1974.

Cobb, S., & Rose, R. Hypertension, peptic ulcer and diabetes in air traffic controllers. *Journal of the American Medical Association*, 1973, *224*, 489–492.

Cofer, C., & Appley, M. *Motivation theory and research*. New York: John Wiley, 1964.

Collea, F. Fate control. Paper presented at the meeting of the California Association of School Psychologists and Psychometrists, Asilomar, Calif., January 12, 1979.

Colligan, M., Smith, J., & Hurrell, J. Occupational incidence rates of mental health disorders. *Journal of Human Stress*, 1977, *3*, 35–39.

Cooper, C., & Marshall, J. The management of stress. *Personnel Review*, 1975, *4*, 27–31.

Cooper, C., & Marshall, J. Occupational sources of stress: A review of the literature relating to coronary heart disease and mental ill health. *Journal of Occupational Psychology* (London), 1976, *49*, 11–28.

Cousins, N. Anatomy of an illness. *Saturday Review*, 1977, *4*, 4–6+.

Davis, K., & Scott, W. *Human relations and organizational behavior: Readings and comments*. New York: McGraw-Hill, 1969.

Dawis, R., Lofquist, L., & Weiss, D. A theory of work adjustment. *Minnesota Studies in Vocational Rehabilitation*, 1968, *23*, 1–31.

Dean, P. Trivial incidents add up to accidents and violence. *San Jose Mercury*, October 23, 1979, p. 2L.

Dickson, W., & Roethlisberger, F. *Management and the worker*. Cambridge, Mass.: Harvard University Press, 1939.

Dohrenwend, B., & Dohrenwend, B. *Stressful life events*. New York: Wiley, 1974.

Downs, C. An empirical and theoretical investigation of communication satisfaction. Paper presented at the meeting of the Speech Communication Association, New York, November 1973.

Dreyfuss, F., & Czackes, J. Blood cholesterol and uric acid of healthy medical students under stress of examination. *Archs Internal Medicine*, 1959, *103*, 705–711.

Dubin, R., Homans, G., Mann, F., & Miller, D. *Leadership and productivity*. San Francisco: Chandler, 1965.

Dyer, W. *Your erroneous zones!* New York: Crowell, 1976.

Eaton, M. The mental health of the older executive. *Geriatrics*, 1969, *24*, 126–134.

Edelfelt, R. The shifting emphasis to inservice teacher education. In Roy Edelfelt (Ed.), *Inservice education: Criteria for and examples of local programs.* Bellingham, Wash.: Western Washington State College, 1977.

Ellis, A. *Humanistic psychotherapy: The rational emotive approach.* New York: Julian Press, 1973.

Erez, M. Feedback: A necessary condition for the goal setting-performance relationship. *Applied Psychology,* 1977, *62,* 624–627.

Felton, J., & Cole, R. The high cost of heart disease. *Circulation,* 1963, *27,* 957–962.

Flesch, R. *Why Johnny can't read and what you can do about it.* New York: Harper & Row, 1966.

Fournet, G., Distefano, M., & Pryer, M. Job satisfaction: Issues and problems. *Personnel Psychology,* 1966, *19,* 165–185.

French, J., & Caplan, R. Psychosocial factors in coronary heart disease. *Industrial Medicine,* 1970, *38,* 383–397.

French, J., & Caplan, R. Organizational stress and individual strain. In A. J. Marrow (Ed.), *The failure of success.* New York, 1973.

Freudenberger, H. Staff burn out. *Journal of Social Issues,* 1974, *30,* 159–165.

Freudenberger, H. The staff burn-out syndrome in alternative institutions. *Psychotherapy: Theory, Research and Practice,* 1975, *12,* 73–82.

Freudenberger, H. The professional and the human services worker: Some solutions to the problems they face in working together. *Journal of Drug Issues,* 1976, *6,* 273–282.

Freudenberger, H. Burn out: Occupational hazard of the child care worker. *Child Care Quarterly,* 1977, *6,* 90–99.

Frew, D. *Management of stress.* Chicago: Nelson Hall, 1977.

Friedman, M. *Pathogenesis of coronary artery disease.* New York: McGraw-Hill, 1969.

Friedman, M., & Rosenman, R. *Type A behavior and your heart.* New York: Knopf, 1974.

Friedman, M., Rosenman, R., & Carroll, V. Changes in serum cholesterol and blood clotting time in men subjected to cyclic variations of occupational stress. *Circulation,* 1958, *17,* 852–861.

Gallup, G. Poll reported at a meeting of the National Association of Secondary School Principals, Las Vegas, February 1975.

Gavin, J., & Axelrod, W. Managerial stress and strain in a mining organization. *Journal of Vocational Behavior,* 1977, *11,* 66–74.

Gechman, A., & Wiener, Y. Job involvement and satisfaction as related to mental health and personal time devoted to work. *Journal of Applied Psychology,* 1975, *60,* 521–523.

Genefore, H. Managerial communication. *Personnel Journal,* 1976, *55,* 568–579.

Gibson, D. Monitoring stress management in the CPI. *Chemical Week,* 1977, *120,* 64–66.

Glass, G., & Smith, M. Class size and student achievement. *Today's Education,* April/May 1979(a), pp. 42–44.

Glass, G., & Smith, M. *Meta-analysis of research on the relationship of class size and achievement.* San Francisco: Far West Laboratory for Educational Research and Development, 1979(b).

Gmelch, W. Beyond stress to effective management. *OSSC Bulletin.* Eugene: University of Oregon, Oregon School Study Council, May/June 1977.

Goleman, D. 1,528 little geniuses and how they grew. *Psychology Today,* February 1980, pp. 29–53.

Greenberg, H. *Coping with job stress.* Englewood Cliffs, N.J.: Prentice-Hall, 1980.

Hasenfeld, Y., & English, R. *Human service organization.* Ann Arbor: University of Michigan Press, 1974.

Hendrickson, B. Principals: Your job is a hazard to your health. *Executive Educator,* March 1979, pp. 22–25, 33.

Herzberg, F. *Motivation to work.* New York: Wiley, 1959.

Herzberg, F. *Work and the nature of man.* New York: World, 1966.

Herzberg, F., Mauser, B., Peterson, R., & Capwell, D. *Job attitudes: Review of research and opinion.* Pittsburgh: Psychological Service, 1957.

Hicks, F. *The mental health of teachers.* New York: Cullman & Ghertner, 1933.

Hollon, C., & Gemmill, G. A comparison of female and male professors on participation in decision making, Job related tension, Job involvement and job satisfaction. *Education Administration Quarterly,* 1976, *12,* 80–93.

Holmes, T., & Rahe, R. The social readjustment rating scale. *Journal of Psychosomatic Research,* 1967, *11,* 213–218.

House, J., & Wells, J. Occupational stress, social support and health. Paper presented at the Conference on Reducing Occupational Stress. New York: National Institute for Occupational Safety and Health Publications, 1977.

How companies cope with executive stress. *Business Week,* August 21, 1978, pp. 107–108.

Howard, J., Rechnitzer, P., & Cunningham, D. Coping with job tension—Effective and ineffective methods. *Public Personnel Management,* 1975, *4,* 317–326.

Huge, J. *Professional burnout.* Englewood, Colo.: Educational Consulting Associates, 1981.

Hulin, C. Effects of changes in job satisfaction levels on employee turnover. *Journal of Applied Psychology,* 1968, *52,* 122–126.

Imberman, W. Letting the employee speak his mind. *Personnel Journal,* 1976, *53,* 12–22.

Jacobson, E. *Progressive relaxation.* Chicago: University of Chicago Press, 1938.

Jacobson, E. *You must relax* (5th ed.). New York: McGraw-Hill, 1978.

Jenkins, C. Psychologic and social precursors of coronary disease. *New England Journal of Medicine,* 1971, *284,* 244–255; 307–319.

Joyce, B., & Morine, G. *Creating the school.* Boston: Little, Brown, 1977.

Joyce, B., & Peck, L. *Inservice teacher education report, interviews.* Syracuse, N.Y.: National Dissemination Center, Syracuse University, 1977.

Joyce, B., Yarger, S., & Howey, K. *Preservice teacher education.* Palo Alto, Calif.: Consolidated Publications, 1977.

Kahn, R. Conflict, ambiguity and overload: Three elements in job stress. *Occupational Mental Health.* 1973, *3,* 2–9.

Kahn, R., & Quinn, R. Role stress. In A. McLean (Ed.), *Mental health and work organization.* Chicago: Rand McNally, 1970.

Kahn, R., Wolfe, D., Quinn, R., Snoek, J., & Rosenthal, R. *Organizational stress: Studies in role conflict and ambiguity.* New York: Wiley, 1964.

Kasl, S. Mental health and work environment: An examination of the evidence. *Journal of Occupational Medicine,* 1973, *15,* 509–518.

Katzell, R. Industrial psychology. In P. Farnsworth & Q. McNemar (Eds.), *Annual Review of Psychology.* Palo Alto, Calif.: Annual Reviews, 1957.

Kearns, J. *Stress in industry.* New York: Priority Press, 1973.

Keninons, G., & Greenhaus, J. Relationship between loss of control and reactions of employees to work characteristics. *Psychological Reports,* 1976, *39,* 815–820.

Kim, J. Effect of feedback on performance and job satisfaction in an organizational setting. Unpublished doctoral dissertation, Michigan State University, 1975.

Kobasa, S., & Maddi, S. Psychological hardiness. *Journal of Occupational Medicine,* 1979, *21,* 595–598.

Koch, J. *Effects of feedback on job attitudes and work behavior* (A Field Experiment, Tech. Rep. 6). University of Oregon, College of Business Administration, Eugene, October 1976.

Kraut, A. A study of role conflicts and their relationships to job satisfaction, tension and performance. Unpublished doctoral dissertation, University of Michigan, 1965.

Kyriacou, C., & Sutcliffe, J. Teacher stress and satisfaction. *Educational Research,* 1975, *21,* 89–96.

Lakein, A. *How to get control of your time and your life.* New York: Peter H. Weyden, 1973.

Lamott, K. *Escape from stress: How to stop killing yourself.* New York: Putnam, 1974.

Lamott, K. *Escape from stress.* New York: Berkeley Medallion, 1975.

LaRocco, J., & Jones, A. Co-worker and leader support as moderators of stress-strain relationships in work situations. *Journal of Applied Psychology,* 1978, *63,* 629–634.

Lawrence, P., & Lorsch, J. *Organization and environment.* New York: Irwin, 1965.

Lazarus, R. *Psychological stress and the coping process.* New York: McGraw-Hill, 1966.

Lee, J., & Shepard, J. Participative management and voluntary turnover: Concepts, theories and implications for management. *National Study Working Papers,* 1972, *71,* 175–193.

Legislative Analyst, State of California. The school principal: A report pursuant to Resolution Chapter 102 of 1977 (ACR 35). Sacramento, October 1977.

Levine, S. Maternal and environmental influences on the adrenocortical response to stress in weaning rats. *Science*, 1967, *156*, 256–258.

Levine, S. Psychosocial factors in growth and development. In L. Levi (Ed.), *Society, stress and disease* (Vol. 2). New York: Oxford University Press, 1975.

Levinson, H. *Executive Stress*. New York: Harper & Row, 1975.

Lieberman, M., & Pearlin, L. Study reported in *Wall Street Journal*, April 2, 1979 ("Age of Anxiety," by J. Bishop), pp. 1, 26.

Lief, H., Fox, R. Training for detached concern in medical students. In H. Lief, V. Lief & N. Lief (Eds.), *The psychological basis of medical practice*. New York: Harper & Row, 1963.

Likert, R. *New patterns of management*. New York: McGraw-Hill, 1961.

Litwak, E. Models of Bureaucracy. *American Journal of Sociology*, 1961, *67*, 177–185.

Locke, E. The nature and causes of job satisfaction. In M. Dunnette (Ed.), *Handbook of industrial and organizational psychology*. Chicago: Rand McNally, 1976.

Luthe, W. *Autogenic therapy, research and theory*. New York: Grune & Stratton, 1970.

McGaffey, T. New horizons in organizational approaches. *Personnel Administration*, 1978, *23*, 26–32.

McGrath, J. A conceptual formulation for research on stress. In J. McGrath (Ed.), *Social and psychological factors in stress*. New York: Holt, Rinehart & Winston, 1970(a).

McGrath, J. *Social and psychological factors in stress*. Chicago: Holt, Rinehart & Winston, 1970(b).

McGregor, D. *The human side of enterprise*. New York: McGraw-Hill, 1960.

McGuire, W. Teacher Burnout. *Today's Education*. 1979, *68*, 5.

McLean, A. (Ed.). *Occupational stress*. Springfield, Ill.: Charles C. Thomas, 1974.

McNally, H. The principalship: A shared responsibility. *National Elementary Principal*, 1975, *55*, 22–28.

Mancuso, J. Executive stress management. *Personnel Administrator*, 1979, *24*, 23–26.

Mangers, D., et. al. *The school principal: Recommendations for effective leadership*. Sacramento, Ca.: California Assembly Education Committee Task Force, 1978.

Manning, D. L. Discontent in the teaching ranks. *Wall Street Journal*, January 9, 1978, p. 12.

Margolis, B., Kroes, W., & Quinn, R. Job stress: An unlisted occupational hazard. *Journal of Occupational Medicine*, 1974(a), *16*, 654–661.

Margolis, B., Kroes, W., & Quinn R. Occupational stress and strain. In A. McLean (Ed.), *Occupational stress*. Springfield, Ill.: Charles C. Thomas, 1974(b).

Martin, L., Roark, A., & Tonso, C. *Participative option development:* Adoption manual (ESEA Title IV). Boulder, Colo.: ESEA, 1978.

Maslach, C. Burned-out. *Human Behavior,* 1976, *5,* 16–22.

Maslach, C. Burn-out: A social psychological analysis. Paper presented at the annual convention of the American Psychological Association, San Francisco, August 1977. To be published in J. W. Jones (Ed.), *The burnout syndrome.* Chicago: London House Press, in press.

Maslach, C., & Pines, A. The burn-out syndrome in the day care setting. *Child Care Quarterly,* 1977, *6,* 100–113.

Mattingly, M. Sources of stress and burn-out in professional child care work. *Child Care Quarterly,* 1977, *6,* 127–137.

Mattox, K. Why teachers quit. *Agricultural Education,* 1974, *49,* 140–142.

Meichenbaum, D. *Cognitive behavior modification.* New York: Plenum Press, 1977.

Miller, J. Information input overload and psychopathology. *American Journal of Psychology,* 1960, *8,* 112–117.

Mintzberg, H. *The nature of managerial work.* San Francisco: Harper & Row, 1973.

Mitchell, D. *Leadership in public education study: A look at the overbooked.* Washington, D.C.: Academy for Education Development, 1972.

Mohrman, A., Cooke, R., & Mohrman, S. Participation in decision making: A multidimensional perspective. *Education Administration Quarterly,* 1978, *14,* 13–29.

Mondale, W. Leave them alone to do their job. *Today's Education,* 1979, *68,* 29.

Morrison, D. Stress and the public administrator. *Public Administration Review,* 1977, *37,* 407–414.

National Association for Mental Health. *Stress at work.* New York: National Association for Mental Health, 1971.

National Education Association. Fit to teach: A study of the health problems of teachers. Washington, D.C.: NEA Department of Classroom Teachers Publications, 1938.

National Education Association. Teaching Load in 1950. *Research Bulletin,* 1951, *29,* 3–50.

National Education Association. Teachers' problems. *Research Bulletin,* 1976, *45,* 116–117.

Neff, W. *Work and human behavior.* New York: Atherton Press, 1968.

New York State Office of Education Performance Review. *School factors influencing reading achievement: A case study of two inner city schools.* New York: Author, 1974.

Nollen, S. Flex time. *Harvard Business Review,* 1979, *57,* 23–28.

Olivero, J. The changing role of the school principal—And what can be done about it. Burlingame, Calif.: Association of California School Administrators Report, February 1979.

Page, R. *How to lick executive stress.* New York: Simon & Schuster, 1966.

Pahl, J., & Pahl, R. *Managers and their wives.* London: Allen Lane, 1971.

Peck, L. A study of the adjustment difficulties of a group of women teachers. *Journal of Educational Psychology*, 1933, *27*, 401–416.

Peterson, K. The principal's task. *Administrators Notebook*, 1978, *26*, 1–9.

Pincherle, G. Fitness for work. *Royal Society of Medicine Journal* (England), 1972, *65*, 321–324.

Porter, L., & Lawler, E. Properties of organization structure in relation to job attitudes and job behavior. *Psychological Bulletin*, 1965, *64*, 23–51.

Pratt, J. Perceived stress among teachers: The effects of age and background of children taught. *Educational Review*, 1978, *30*, 3–14.

Pritchard, R., & Montagno, R. Effects of specific vs. nonspecific and absolute vs. comparative feedback on performance and satisfaction. *Purdue Research Foundation Report.* Lafayette, Ind.: May 1978.

Proctor, P. How to survive today's stressful jobs. *Parade Magazine*, June 17, 1979.

Puff, H., & Moeckel, C. Managerial stress and the woman manager. *Industrial Management*, 1979, *21*, 1–5.

Quick, J., & Quick, J. Reducing stress through preventative management. *Human Resource Management*, 1979, *18*, 15–22.

Quinn, R., Seashore, S., & Mangione, I. *Survey of working conditions.* Washington, D.C.: U.S. Government Printing Office, 1971.

Reed, S. What can you do to prevent teacher burnout. *National Elementary Principal*, 1979, *58*, 66–71.

Roark, A., & Davis, W. Staff development and organization development. In Betty Dillon-Peterson (Ed.), *Staff development/organizational development.* Alexandria, Va.: Association for Supervision and Curriculum Development, 1980.

Rogers, R. Executive stress. *Human Resource Management*, 1975, *14*, 21–24.

Rogers, R. Components of organizational stress among Canadian managers. *Journal of Psychology*, 1977, *95*, 265–273.

Ross, I., & Zander, A. Need satisfactions and employee turnover. *Personnel Psychology*, 1957, *10*, 327–338.

Rosten, L. "The free mind." Speech delivered at 1962 National Book Awards. Quoted in *Washington Post*, 1962. Cited in L. Rosten, *The Many Worlds of Leo Rosten.* New York: Harper & Row, 1964, pp. 203–209.

Rubin, L. The case for staff development. In Thomas Sergiovanni (Ed.), *Professional supervision for professional teachers.* Alexandria, Va.: Association for Supervision and Curriculum Development, 1975.

Ruch, W., Hershauer, J., & Wright, R. Toward solving the productivity puzzle: Worker correlates to performance. *Human Resource Management*, 1976, *15*, 2–6.

Ryan, W. *Blaming the victim.* New York: Vintage, 1971.

Sales, S. Some effects of role overload and role underload. *Organizational Behavior and Human Performance*, 1970, *5*, 592–608.

Sarason, S., Sarason, E., & Cowden, P. Aging and the nature of work. *American Psychologist*, 1975, *30*, 584–593.

Schafer, W. *Stress, distress and growth*. Davis, Calif.: Responsible Action Publication, 1978.

Schwartz, D. Health status assessment. In A. McLean (Ed.), *Occupational stress*. Springfield, Ill.: Charles C. Thomas, 1974.

Seashore, S. Group cohesiveness in the industrial work group. Ann Arbor: University of Michigan Institute for Social Research, 1954.

Seligmann, J., & Huck, J. Burnt-out principals. *Newsweek*, March 19, 1978.

Selye, H. *Stress without distress*. New York: Lippincott, 1974.

Selye, H. *The stress of life* (2nd ed.). New York: McGraw-Hill, 1976.

Selye, H. Stress without distress (synopsis). *The school guidance worker* (Toronto), 1977, 5, 5–13.

Shealley, C. *Ninety days to self health*. New York: Bantam, 1977.

Shirom, A., Eden, D., Silberwasser, S., & Kellerman, J. Job stresses and risk factors in coronary heart disease among occupational categories in kibbutzim. *Social Science Medical*, 1973, 7, 875–892.

Simpe, J. Job strain as a function of job and life stresses. Unpublished doctoral dissertation, Colorado State University, 1975.

Sommers, D. Burnout. *Inc.*, December 1980, pp. 57–58, 60, 62.

Spaniol, L., & Caputo, J. *Professional burn-out: A personal survival kit*. Lexington, Mass.: Human Services Associates, 1979.

Sparks, D. A biased look at teacher job satisfaction. *Clearing House*, 1979, 52, 447–491.

Stoyva, J. A psychophysiological model of stress disorders as a rationale for biofeedback training. In F. McGuigan (Ed.), *Tension control: Proceedings of the second meeting of the American Society for the Advancement of Tension Control*. Blacksburg, Va.: University Publications, 1976.

Stress on teachers and other school personnel (National Education Association Resolution E 79–81). *Today's Education*, November/December 1979, p. 36.

Stull, J. Educator evaluations (Report made to the California State Senate). Sacramento, Calif., November 1978.

Suinn, R. How to break the vicious cycle of stress. *Psychology Today*, December 1976, pp. 59–60.

Tannenbaum, A. Control in organizations: Individual adjustment and organizational performance. *Administrative Science Quarterly*, 1962, 7, 236–257.

Teacher burnout. *Wall Street Journal*, July 25, 1979(a), p. 20.

Teacher burnout: How to cope when your world goes black. *Instructor*, 1979(b), 88, 56–62.

Teacher burnout: A national issue says NEA panel. *NEA Reporter*, October 1979(c), p. 7.

Terhune, W. Emotional problems of executives in time. *Industrial Medicine and Surgery*, 1963, 32, 1–67.

Terryberry, S. *The organization of environments*. Unpublished doctoral dissertation, University of Michigan, 1968.

Thompson, P., & Dalton, G. Are R&D organizations obsolete? *Harvard Business Review,* November/December 1976, pp. 105–116.

Thompson, V. Bureaucracy and innovation. *Administrative Science Quarterly,* 1965, *10,* 1–20.

Truch, S. *Teacher burnout.* Novato, Calif.: Academic Therapy Publications, 1980.

Vail, D. *Dehumanization and the institutional career.* Springfield, Ill.: Charles C. Thomas, 1966.

Vetter, E. Role pressure and the school principal. *NASSP Bulletin,* 1976, *60,* 11–23.

Vroom, V. *Some personality determinants of the effects of participation.* Englewood Cliffs, N.J.: Prentice-Hall, 1960.

Vroom, V. *Work and motivation.* New York: Wiley, 1964.

Wagstaff, L. Unionized principals—You may be next. *NASSP Bulletin,* 1973, *57,* 40–47.

Wahlund, I., & Nerell, G. *Stress factors in the working environments of white collar workers.* Chicago: National Institute of Safety and Health, 1977.

Wardwell, W., Hyman, M., & Bahnson, C. Stress and coronary heart disease in three field studies. *Journal of Chronic Disease,* 1970, *22,* 781–795.

Weber, M. *Essays in sociology.* Edited and translated by H. Gerth and C. W. Mills. New York: Oxford University Press, 1946.

Weitzel, W., Pinto, P., Dawis, R., & Jury, R. The impact of the organization on the structure of job satisfaction: Some path analytic findings. *Personnel Psychology,* 1973, *26,* 545–557.

West, N. How chief executives handle stress. *Los Angeles Business and Economics,* Winter 1978, pp. 6–11.

Wickert, R. Turnover and employees' feelings of ego-involvement in the day to day operation of a company. *Personnel Psychology,* 1951, *4,* 185–197.

Wilson, C. Patterns of teacher stress. Survey conducted in San Diego County, San Diego, Calif.: Department of Education, 1979.

Withall, J., & Wood, F. Taking the threat out of classroom observation and feedback. *Journal of Teacher Education,* 1979, *30,* 55–58.

Wood, F., Thompson, S., & Russell, F. Designing effective staff development programs. In B. Dillon-Peterson (Ed.), *Staff development/organization development.* Alexandria, Va.: Association for Supervision and Curriculum Development, 1981, pp. 59–91.

Index